Complications in Breast Reduction

Editor

DENNIS C. HAMMOND

CLINICS IN PLASTIC SURGERY

www.plasticsurgery.theclinics.com

April 2016 • Volume 43 • Number 2

ELSEVIER

1600 John F. Kennedy Boulevard • Suite 1800 • Philadelphia, Pennsylvania, 19103-2899

http://www.theclinics.com

CLINICS IN PLASTIC SURGERY Volume 43, Number 2
April 2016 ISSN 0094-1298, ISBN-13: 978-0-323-44283-1

Editor: Jessica McCool
Developmental Editor: Donald Mumford

Clinics in Plastic Surgery (ISSN 0094-1298) is published quarterly by Elsevier Inc., 360 Park Avenue South, New York, NY 10010-1710. Months of issue are January, April, July, and October. Business and Editorial Offices: 1600 John F. Kennedy Blvd., Suite 1800, Philadelphia, PA 19103-2899. Periodicals postage paid at New York, NY and additional mailing offices. Subscription prices are $490.00 per year for US individuals, $793.00 per year for US institutions, $100.00 per year for US students and residents, $555.00 per year for Canadian individuals, $944.00 per year for Canadian institutions, $630.00 per year for international individuals, $944.00 per year for international institutions, and $305.00 per year for Canadian and foreign students/residents. To receive student/resident rate, orders must be accompanied by name of affiliated institution, date of term, and the *signature* of program/residency coordinator on institution letterhead. Orders will be billed at individual rate until proof of status is received. Foreign air speed delivery is included in all *Clinics* subscription prices. All prices are subject to change without notice. **POSTMASTER:** Send address changes to *Clinics in Plastic Surgery*, Elsevier Health Sciences Division, Subscription Customer Service, 3251 Riverport Lane, Maryland Heights, MO 63043. **Customer Service: 1-800-654-2452 (US and Canada). From outside of the United States and Canada, call 314-447-8871. Fax: 314-447-8029. E-mail:** JournalsCustomerService-usa@elsevier.com **(for print support);** JournalsOnlineSupport-usa@elsevier.com **(for online support).**

Reprints. For copies of 100 or more of articles in this publication, please contact the Commercial Reprints Department, Elsevier Inc., 360 Park Avenue South, New York, New York 10010-1710. Tel.: +1-212-633-3874; Fax: +1-212-633-3820; E-mail: reprints@elsevier.com.

Clinics in Plastic Surgery is covered in *Current Contents, EMBASE/Excerpta Medica, Science Citation Index, MEDLINE/PubMed (Index Medicus), ASCA,* and *ISI/BIOMED.*

Contributors

EDITOR

DENNIS C. HAMMOND, MD
Assistant Program Director, Plastic Surgery
Residency, Grand Rapids Area Medical
Education Partners, Partners in Plastic
Surgery, Grand Rapids, Michigan

AUTHORS

JAMIL AHMAD, MD, FRCSC
Assistant Professor, Division of Plastic and
Reconstructive Surgery, University of Toronto,
Toronto, Ontario, Canada

FRANK P. ALBINO, MD
Department of Plastic Surgery, MedStar
Georgetown University Hospital,
Washington, DC

CLAUDIO ANGRIGIANI, MD
Department of Oncoplastic Surgery, Instituto
Oncologico Henry Moore, University of Buenos
Aires, Argentina

RYAN E. AUSTIN, MD
Chief Resident, Division of Plastic and
Reconstructive Surgery, University of Toronto,
Toronto, Ontario, Canada

GRANT W. CARLSON, MD
Wadley R. Glenn Professor of Surgery, Chief of
the Division of Plastic Surgery; Department of
Surgery, School of Medicine, Emory University,
Atlanta, Georgia

**EDWARD H. DAVIDSON, MA (Cantab),
MBBS**
Chief Resident, Department of Plastic Surgery,
University of Pittsburgh, Pittsburgh,
Pennsylvania

ALBERT DE MEY, MD
Honorary Professor, Plastic Surgery, Free
University Brussels; Clinique du Parc Léopold,
Brussels, Belgium

ONELIO GARCIA Jr, MD, FACS
Vol. Assistant Professor, Division
of Plastic Surgery, University of Miami, Miller
School of Medicine, Miami, Florida

JEFFREY A. GUSENOFF, MD
Associate Professor, Department of Plastic
Surgery, University of Pittsburgh, Pittsburgh,
Pennsylvania

DENNIS C. HAMMOND, MD
Assistant Program Director, Plastic Surgery
Residency, Grand Rapids Area Medical
Education Partners, Partners in Plastic
Surgery, Grand Rapids, Michigan

PRIYANKA HANDA, MD
Division of Plastic and Reconstructive Surgery,
Department of Radiology, Emory University,
Atlanta, Georgia

NEAL HANDEL, MD, FACS
Associate Clinical Professor, Division of Plastic
Surgery, Geffen School of Medicine at
University of California Los Angeles,
Los Angeles, California

JULIANA E. HANSEN, MD
Professor and Chief, Plastic and
Reconstructive Surgery, Department of
Surgery, Oregon Health and Science
University, Portland, Oregon

MARCELO IRIGO, MD, PhD
Department of Oncoplastic Surgery,
Instituto Oncologico Henry Moore,
University of Buenos Aires, Argentina

KUYLHEE KIM, MD
Partners in Plastic Surgery, Grand Rapids, Michigan

RUSSELL E. KLING, MD
Resident, Department of Plastic Surgery, University of Pittsburgh, Pittsburgh, Pennsylvania

FRANK LISTA, MD, FRCSC
Assistant Professor, Division of Plastic and Reconstructive Surgery, University of Toronto, Toronto, Ontario, Canada

ALBERT LOSKEN, MD
Division of Plastic and Reconstructive Surgery, Emory University, Atlanta, Georgia

MARTA MISANI, MD
Plastic Surgeon, CHR Mons Hainaut, Mons, Belgium

MARY S. NEWELL, MD
Division of Plastic and Reconstructive Surgery, Department of Radiology, Emory University, Atlanta, Georgia

YAN T. ORTIZ-POMALES, MD, FACS
Division of Plastic and Reconstructive Surgery, Emory University, Atlanta, Georgia

LINDA G. PHILLIPS, MD
Professor and Chief, Division of Plastic Surgery, Department of Surgery, University of Texas Medical Branch, Galveston, Texas

KAREN L. POWERS, MD
Section of Plastic Surgery, Department of Surgery, Lakeland Regional Medical Center, St. Joseph, Michigan

ALBERTO RANCATI, MD, PhD
Department of Oncoplastic Surgery, Instituto Oncologico Henry Moore, University of Buenos Aires, Argentina

NEAL R. REISMAN, MD, JD, FACS
Attorney at Law; Chief, Plastic Surgery, Baylor-St. Luke's Hospital; Clinical Professor of Plastic Surgery, Baylor College of Medicine, Houston, Texas

J. PETER RUBIN, MD, FACS
Chair, Department of Plastic Surgery; University of Pittsburgh Medical Center Endowed Professor of Plastic Surgery; Professor of Bioengineering, University of Pittsburgh, Pittsburgh, Pennsylvania

KENNETH C. SHESTAK, MD
Professor and Chief, Department of Plastic Surgery, Magee Womens Hospital, University of Pittsburgh, Pittsburgh, Pennsylvania

SCOTT L. SPEAR, MD
Private Practice, Washington, DC

WILLIAM D. TOBLER Jr, MD
Resident, Department of Plastic Surgery, University of Pittsburgh, Pittsburgh, Pennsylvania

SARA YEGIYANTS, MD
Division of Plastic Surgery, Geffen School of Medicine at University of California Los Angeles, Los Angeles, California

Contents

Assessing risk and avoiding complications in breast reduction requires a meticulous history, systematic physical examination, management of expectations, and careful consideration and execution of operative technique. Attention should be paid to co-morbidities. Shape, symmetry, contours, scar location, skin quality, nipple–areolar complex (NAC) shape, NAC position relative to inframammary fold, and NAC position relative to the volume of the breast should be evaluated. Because complications cannot always be anticipated, informed consent is a vital part of managing expectations. Intraoperative considerations include blood pressure control, limiting tension, delayed healing and tissue loss, and using applied anatomy to avoid malposition and asymmetry.

Breast reduction surgery is one of the most popular procedures performed by plastic surgeons; based on the current literature, it is safe and does not have a negative impact on identifying breast cancer in women. There are no evidence-based data to confirm the utility of unique screening protocols for women planning to undergo reduction surgery or for those who already had reduction. Women undergoing this surgery should not deviate from the current recommendations of screening mammography in women older than 40 years of average risk. Experienced radiologists can readily distinguish postsurgical imaging findings of rearranged breast parenchyma from malignancy.

The incidence of occult breast cancer detected by reduction mammaplasty is 0.06% to 5.45%. Preoperative screening mammography is indicated in all women 40 years and older and in women age 35 with a positive family or personal history of breast cancer before reduction mammaplasty. Breast MRI is considered in women with dense breasts and those with hereditary breast cancer syndromes. Management of occult breast cancer is impacted by specimens being typically removed in pieces and not oriented before submission to pathology. Total mastectomy is the most common treatment because of the uncertainties regarding margin status and disease extent.

Wise pattern breast reduction remains the most popular method of performing moderate- to large-sized breast reductions in the United States. Shape distortion after breast reduction can be a result of design flaw, execution of technique, or the result of postoperative complications. This article focuses primarily on optimal design and intraoperative techniques for prevention of shape distortion. By carefully considering the design of the skin resection pattern, choosing and designing an appropriate pedicle, preventing skin necrosis, and managing scars, shape distortion after Wise pattern breast reduction can be minimized.

In this paper, we describe our experience with the Lejour vertical scar mammaplasty from its description throughout 25 years of practice. Our work aims to focus on reducing vertical scar mammaplasty complications by examining results, studying how to avoid unfavorable consequences, and providing new tips to improve the technique and shorten its learning curve. Complications can be related to patient characteristics and habits, but adhering to a strict surgical protocol is essential to limit other factors. The importance of recognizing and being able to manage the complications is mandatory to have a successful final result and a satisfied patient.

Breast reduction is one of the most common plastic surgery procedures performed on the breast. There are now numerous alternatives to the standard inverted-T inferior pedicle technique. The short scar periareolar inferior pedicle reduction (SPAIR) mammaplasty is one of these techniques. The procedure was designed to reduce the scar burden associated with breast reduction. However, postoperative complications can occur. The purpose of this article is to outline these potential complications that are of particular concern with the SPAIR mammaplasty and describe methods for their treatment and prevention.

Breast reduction surgery has achieved one of the highest patient satisfaction rates among plastic surgery procedures. Most of the complications encountered are usually minor and related to wound healing. Revision surgery to address these problems is common and usually consists of scar revisions. Postoperative breast asymmetry of a mild degree is also common; however, postoperative asymmetry severe enough to warrant surgical revision is a rare event, occurring in less than 1% of cases. Post-mammaplasty revision surgery needs to be individualized. The asymmetry could be the result of nipple malposition or it could consist of a volume or shape discrepancy between the breast mounds.

Recurrent or persistent macromastia can occur after breast reduction. This may be due to inadequate primary volume reduction, poor postoperative shape, and breast or nipple-areola complex asymmetry. Postpartum breast changes, weight change, and aging can also contribute to recurrent macromastia. The concern in these cases is the altered blood supply to the nipple-areola complex and the safety of nipple-areola complex transposition. Literature on the safety of repeated breast reduction is limited with conflicting approaches. This article discusses an approach to recurrent or persistent macromastia and outlines a modified breast reduction technique that is safe in cases of repeated breast reduction.

unburned breasts. The extent of the deformity, the location of the deformity, and the status of the surrounding soft tissue are all assessed before embarking on any surgical plan, which then proceeds in a conservative stepwise fashion. Although many plastic surgeons are reluctant to operate on burned breasts for fear of devascularizing the skin graft or nipple areolar complex, reduction mammaplasty in this group of patients is safe and carries minimal risk if key concepts are followed.

Gigantomastia is a disabling condition for patients and presents unique challenges to plastic surgeons. Presentation can occur throughout different phases of life, and treatment often begins with nonoperative measures; however, the most effective way to relieve symptoms is surgical breast reduction. Because of the large amount of tissue removed, surgeons can encounter different intraoperative and postoperative complications. By understanding this disease process and these complications, surgeons can attempt to minimize their occurrences. The authors present an overview of the cause, preoperative evaluation, techniques, and outcomes. Additionally, they present outcomes data from their center on 40 patients.

Areas of general risk are discussed with patients before surgery. Procedure-specific risks inherent in each technique are a key part of informed consent. Issues related to insurance coverage must be settled preoperatively to decrease litigation risk. Protection of patient information has become a key part of the overall treatment process and this information must be protected.

CLINICS IN PLASTIC SURGERY

THE CLINICS ARE AVAILABLE ONLINE!
Access your subscription at:
www.theclinics.com

Preface
Complications in Plastic Surgery

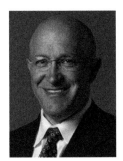

Dennis C. Hammond, MD
Editor

Breast reduction is one of the most commonly performed procedures in plastic surgery, and many different techniques have been described to accomplish this task. However, concentrated information on the management of complications associated with this workhorse operation is lacking. This was the impetus for this issue of *Clinics in Plastic Surgery*. The content is organized into four subcategories, including (1) general considerations in breast reduction and management of issues related to breast cancer; (2) specific discussion of complication management for each of the common techniques in breast reduction; (3) management of specific complications common to all techniques and management of specific difficult types of patients; and (4) management of medicolegal issues related to breast reduction. Each of the authors is a recognized expert in plastic surgery of the breast, and I would specifically like to extend my sincere gratitude for their efforts in making this a highlight issue of this very respected series, *Clinics in Plastic Surgery*. It is my hope that you, the reader, will find this information useful in the management of your own patients.

Dennis C. Hammond, MD
Partners in Plastic Surgery
4070 Lake Drive, Suite 202
Grand Rapids, MI 49546, USA

E-mail address:
drhammond@pipsmd.com

Clin Plastic Surg 43 (2016) xi
http://dx.doi.org/10.1016/j.cps.2016.01.001
0094-1298/16/$ – see front matter © 2016 Published by Elsevier Inc.

Assessing Risk and Avoiding Complications in Breast Reduction

Kenneth C. Shestak, MD[a,b,*], Edward H. Davidson, MA (Cantab), MBBS[a]

KEYWORDS

- Breast reduction • Complications • Preoperative assessment • Scar
- Nipple areola complex (NAC) malposition • Delayed wound healing • Skin loss • Asymmetry

KEY POINTS

- A thorough history and physical examination are fundamental in identifying patients at greater risk of complications after breast reduction and to guide risk reduction and planning.
- Perioperative optimization and lifestyle modulation to mitigate risk, as well as technical considerations in preoperative planning and execution, can help to avoid complications.
- Patient-appropriate technique selection and understanding of technical principles of breast reduction can help to avoid surgical complications.
- Some patients experience complications; preoperative explanation of this should be part of the informed consent process, which helps in managing patient expectations for the procedure.
- Overall, complications of breast reduction surgery are well-tolerated by patients, who are usually satisfied if their symptoms of macromastia are relieved.

INTRODUCTION

The surgical goal of breast reduction is the removal of breast tissue to treat the symptoms of macromastia. An ideal breast reduction surgery should also produce symmetric, well-shaped breasts with well-positioned, sensate nipple–areolar complexes (NACs). Furthermore, these results should have longevity and be achieved with an acceptable scar trade off.

Complications of breast reduction surgery include those that are inherent to any surgery, that is, things that affect the way a wound heals. In addition, there are anesthesia-related risks, for example, deep vein thrombosis and pulmonary embolism.

There are also those that are not systemic, but rather plastic surgical complications related to the surgery of breast itself and the way this paired organ looks after surgery. This article focuses on the assessment of risk and avoidance of these complications. Such complications maybe acute, subacute, or long term (**Box 1**).[1] Delayed wound healing is usually cited as the most common complication (**Box 2**).[2]

A meticulous history and examination are necessary to assess the risk of these complications as well as careful operative planning and technical considerations to avoid them. Complications cannot always be avoided; said another way, only the surgeon who does not operate has no

Disclosure Statement: K. C. Shestak receives royalties from Lippincott Williams & Wilkins for reoperative plastic surgery of the breast. K. C Shestak 2006; Dr Shestak has also served on an Advisory Board of Allergan Medical Corp; E. H. Davidson has nothing to disclose.
[a] Department of Plastic Surgery, University of Pittsburgh, 3550 Terrace Street, 6B Scaife Hall, Pittsburgh, PA 15213, USA; [b] Department of Plastic Surgery, Magee Womens Hospital, 3380 Boulevard of Allies Suite 180, Pittsburgh, PA 15213, USA
* Corresponding author. Department of Plastic Surgery, Magee Womens Hospital, 3380 Boulevard of Allies Suite 180, Pittsburgh, PA 15213.
E-mail address: shestakkc@upmc.edu

plasticsurgery.theclinics.com

Box 1
Complications of breast reduction

Acute Complications	Subacute Complications	Long-Term Complications
Hematoma	Asymmetry	Contour deformities
Seroma	Hypertrophic scars	Recurrent ptosis
Skin loss	Fat necrosis	Scar deformities/unfavorable scars
Wound separation		Loss of shape
Cellulitis		Nipple malposition
Nipple areola ischemia		Underresection
		Overresection
		Inability to breast feed
		Failure to resolve symptoms of macromastia

From Shestak KC. Re-operative plastic surgery of the breast. Philadelphia: Lippincott Williams & Wilkins; 2006; with permission.

Box 2
Complications of breast reduction by incidence

Complication	Incidence (%)
Delayed wound healing	21.6
Spitting sutures	9.2
Hematoma	3.7
Nipple necrosis	3.6
Hypertrophic scars	2.5
Fat necrosis	1.8
Seroma	1.2
Infection	1.2

Key Elements of History to Assess for Risk of Breast Reduction Complications

Patient symptoms and expectations
Comorbidities (including diabetes, hypertension, coagulopathy, connective tissue disorders, obesity)
Previous hypertrophic scarring/keloids
Smoking habits
Obstetric history
Medications
Mammogram status

Key Elements of Physical Examination to Assess for Risk of Breast Reduction Complications

Shape
Symmetry
Contours
Scar location
Skin quality and elasticity
NAC shape
NAC position relative to IMF
NAC position relative to the volume of the breast
Volume distribution of both skin and parenchyma.
Specific measurements (suprasternal notch to nipple distance, breast base width, Nipple to IMF distance, Nipple to midline distance)
Estimated volume of resection

Abbreviations: IMF, inframammary fold; NAC, nipple–areola complex.

From Cunningham BL, Gear AJ, Kerrigan CL, et al. Analysis of breast reduction complications derived from the BRAVO study. Plast Reconstr Surg 2005;115(6):1597–604; with permission.

complications (anonymous; but quoted by many experienced surgeons). Nonetheless, identification of those patients at relatively greater risk enables the surgeon to optimize these patients preoperatively. Although it is not always possible to eliminate complications, preoperatively educating patients and counseling them appropriately, with full disclosure of these risks as part of an informed consenting process, is vital in managing expectations for a patient who chooses to pursue surgery with a potential benefit that may outweigh the risk or reality of a complication.

ASSESSMENT OF RISK HISTORY

As with all operations, an understanding of the primary complaint(s) of the patient is necessary. Patients must have symptomatic macromastia to undergo breast reduction surgery, because fundamentally this is a "functional" surgical intervention aimed at addressing these symptoms. Specific symptoms may include back pain, neck, pain, rashes/skin irritation, and bra strap grooving. These symptoms should be probed to ensure there is no other etiology aside from the breast that is the cause. If the patient is not significantly burdened by this symptomatology or if symptoms are not owing to macromastia, then reduction mammaplasty may not result in an optimal outcome but rather an unsatisfied patient. Surgery in the absence of symptoms, but merely to address a patient's size concerns requires a careful discussion of the "tradeoff of size and shape for scars" to ensure a patient's expectations are appropriately managed.

Particular attention must be paid to past medical history. A history of hypertrophic scarring or keloids risks this occurring after breast reduction; connective tissue disorders risks delayed wound healing; diabetes increases risk of infection; hypercoagulopathy (which may be suggested by multiple spontaneous abortions or miscarriages) may increase risk of thromboembolic complications or bleeding/hematoma, as can hypertension; and a prior methicillin-resistant *Staphylococcus aureus* infection or similar can also increase risk of infective complications. In each instance, preoperative optimization must be ensured; otherwise, complications should be anticipated.

The impact of obesity on complications in breast reduction surgery remains unclear. The overall complication rate has been shown by some to be greater in obese patients with increased rates of delayed healing, seroma, infection, skin and/or nipple–areola necrosis, hematoma, fat necrosis, stitch abscesses, diminished nipple sensation, and hypertrophic scarring.[2–9] However, studies have failed to show this consistently. Analysis of complication data derived from the Breast Reduction Assessment: Value and Outcomes (BRAVO) study, a 9-month prospective, multicenter trial, demonstrated no relation between obesity and complications after breast reduction. Although breast reduction has been shown to be safe in the morbidly obese, careful consideration is needed in the decision over breast reduction in morbidly obese patients, who often have other major health problems, including increased anesthesia-related risk. In any event, the health benefits of breast reduction surgery in these patients are long term and may far exceed the risks of local complications.[10,11]

An additional important factor is smoking. The perioperative morbidity associated with ongoing smoking is well-established. In breast reduction, specifically, there is an abundance of evidence to support an increased complication rate among smokers in the region of 3-fold that of non-smokers.[2,12–14] The cessation time period necessary to prevent wound healing complications is not known. In the absence of research-proven guidelines concerning smoking and elective surgery, a wide variability of treatment algorithms have been developed among individual surgeons. A common recommendation is a 4-week period of no smoking both before and after surgery. If the surgeon suspects noncompliance, a urine nicotinine test is recommended by many surgeons preoperatively and can detect if a patient has smoked within the last 4 days.[14,15]

Obtaining an accurate obstetric history is also important in these patients. As alluded to, a history of miscarriage may suggest an underlying coagulopathy. From a more commonly encountered empiric perspective, breast size most often enlarges with pregnancy. Therefore, if the patient is planning for children in the near future then consideration of delaying until planned pregnancies are completed might be prudent to ultimately ensure a desirable surgical outcome. Similarly, given the uncertainty regarding the possible negative impact on breast feeding performance of reduction mammaplasty, to avoid disappointment and inability to breast feed, delaying surgery until after nursing should be a consideration.[16–19] On a related issue, patients desiring breast reduction surgery over the age of 40 should have had a mammogram within the last year given the incidence of occult breast cancer in breast reduction specimens is 0.06% to 0.4%.[20]

A careful review of a patient's medications is necessary. Nonsteroidal antiinflammatory drugs including aspirin and ibuprofen, as well as herbal supplements and prescribed anticoagulants, increase bleeding risk. Oral contraceptives are associated with thrombosis and can increase the risk slightly. Steroids can impair wound healing. This is by no means an exhaustive list but demonstrative of the importance of appropriate awareness and planning for perioperative medication management.

ASSESSMENT OF RISK: PHYSICAL EXAMINATION

A full and systematic examination of the breasts is mandatory for the assessment of risk of complication in breast reduction. On inspection, the following should be assessed: shape, symmetry, contours, scar location, skin quality, NAC shape, NAC position relative to inframammary fold (IMF), and NAC position relative to the volume of the breast. The presence of prominent lateral chest rolls that are not part of the breast is very common and should be noted and demonstrated to the patient. Typically, these would not be addressed by standard reduction mammaplasty techniques and will remain postoperatively. However, they can be addressed concomitantly with liposuction and limited excision under a "fee-for-service" format if the patient so desires.

Specific measurements of breast topography and anatomic landmarks should also be made. These most commonly include the suprasternal notch to nipple distance, breast base width, nipple to IMF distance, and nipple to midline distance. In addition, anteroposterior, oblique and lateral photographs also allow for later study to aid in operative planning. Palpation for any masses or scars should be performed along with tactile examination of the quality, elasticity, and volume distribution of both the skin and the parenchyma.

The importance of these analyses in predicting risk is in the identification of gross asymmetries, an appreciation of the volume of resection and assessment of pedicle length, and potential for loss of NAC viability. It is part of surgical planning to address such asymmetries; designing incision pattern and resection to attempt to better harmonize the breasts with respect to one another. Objective identification of asymmetry also allows the surgeon to council the patient in a more demonstrative way. In this manner, patients can appreciate asymmetries may remain after surgery, and may even be more apparent (even if objectively they are improved) when they are no longer "masked" by the excess of breast volume.

Estimating the volume of resection has ramifications for candidacy for the procedure, both in terms of therapeutic benefit and insurance coverage, as well as possibly being a predictor for surgical complications. Patients who do not fulfill the criteria for reduction surgery (bra cup less than size D, estimated excess of breast tissue less than 400 g, and equivocal symptomatology) are counseled not to pursue breast reduction surgery. If the estimated excess of tissue is less than 400 g and sufficient ptosis is present, the patient may be a far better candidate for a cosmetic mastopexy. It should be noted that patients with at least 400 g excess on 1 side and significant breast asymmetry (greater than 1 cup size) may qualify for breast reduction. Exceptions also are made for patients less than 18 years of age if their symptoms are severe and they demonstrate a clear understanding of the risks of surgery.[21]

Controversy exists in the literature regarding whether volume of resection is an independent risk factor for surgical complications. In part, this controversy exists owing to the difficulty in isolating this from the confounders of any coexisting obesity and technique used. A 10-year review of nearly 400 patients determined patients who undergo resections of greater than 1200 g would be expected to have a complication rate approximately 5 times greater than patients with resections of less than 300 g and approximately 3 times greater than patients with the most frequently performed resection of 300 to 600 g. Reports in the literature have suggested that the cause of complications in a larger breast is long pedicle length associated with the inferior pedicle technique. Although this may be true, this may not be the only reason, because this study found that the correlation also held true for the free nipple graft patients.[6] Analysis of breast reduction complications derived from the BRAVO study found that delayed wound healing, the most common complication, correlated directly with average preoperative breast volume and average resection weight. Logistic regression analysis associated resection weight as the sole variable for increased risk of complications. Each 10-fold increase in resection weight increased the risk of complication 4.8 times and increased the risk of delayed healing 11.6 times.[2]

Measurements of suprasternal notch to nipple distance, breast base width, nipple to IMF distance, and nipple to midline distance allow the surgeon to estimate pedicle length of the various breast reduction techniques. For example, nipple to IMF distance is analogous to the pedicle length in an inferior pedicle technique. Undoubtedly, one of the most significant complications of reduction mammaplasty is vascular compromise of the nipple. Although this may be less of a problem if the bulk of the pedicle is increased, it has been stated that the length of the pedicle is the most important criterion for decision making, and this is the measurement that should be the basis for the decision whether a pedicle technique or a free nipple graft is to be used.[22] The question of how long is too long for a pedicle cannot be definitively answered with an arbitrary number. In the senior author's experience, for the inferior pedicle technique a pedicle length of up to 20 cm can produce nipple viability in most cases. A surgeon's judgment, as well as balancing patient expectations regarding NAC form and function with the comorbidities of the prolonged procedure, can determine preoperatively whether to pursue pedicle-based breast reduction versus breast tissue resection (amputation technique) and nipple grafting. In 'borderline' cases, patients should be consented that a pedicled procedure may require conversion to nipple grafting based on intraoperative findings.

AVOIDANCE OF COMPLICATIONS: GENERAL CONSIDERATIONS

With a thorough history and physical examination outlined, risk of complications after reduction mammaplasty may be mitigated, where possible, with lifestyle modification and perioperative medical optimization. There are patients who nonetheless will be of relatively higher risk. To some degree, operative planning can decrease this risk, especially of more major complications such as nipple loss. However, some patients will have complications; some will have unsightly scarring, some will develop seroma, some will have delayed healing and surgical site infections will occur. The key to managing complications is therefore not just to anticipate and evolve the surgical plan where possible (although this is essential), but rather to manage expectations. The role of the responsible surgeon is not just to deliver a safe and efficacious procedure in the operating room, but also to transfer their body of knowledge to the patient such that they understand the possible outcomes preoperatively and thus consent to a procedure in an informed way. Describing the course of potential complications and their management, showing photographs of representative results and scars, and so on allows the patient to appreciate surgery not simply as an "event," but rather a process in which adversity may occur and as such may not even be perceived as a complication per se. Finally and importantly, the surgeon must convey that he or she will be there to help the patent through postoperative problems if they occur.

AVOIDANCE OF COMPLICATIONS: TECHNIQUE SELECTION

The merits of the various techniques for breast reduction are discussed elsewhere. Although training bias and experience do play a role, it is often difficult for the plastic surgeon choosing a technique for breast reduction to decide what surgical procedure will serve the patient best. In general terms, some techniques are more suited to some patients than others. For example, both vertical pattern and Wise pattern techniques have advantages and disadvantages. The standard Wise pattern resection with an inferiorly based pedicle is easy to perform and reliable, all skin excess is removed, and the breast has good conical shape at the completion of the procedure. The disadvantages are that it results in an inverted T scar that might be objectionable to some patients, and it might have poor long-term shape owing to bottoming out. In contrast, the vertical reduction mammaplasty results in only periareolar and vertical scars with the promise of improved shape. However, in large breasts the redundant skin in the lower pole can often form a "dog ear" that takes a protracted time to "settle" or requires a surgical revision.[23] In general, smaller and moderate sized breast reductions may be amenable to a vertical pattern technique whereas relatively larger reductions are best achieved with less risk of complications by means of a Wise pattern technique.

There are controversies regarding which pedicle is the most reliable concerning vasculature and shape. Vascular variability and overlap may account for the remarkable safety of diverse NAC–bearing pedicles, even though pedicle thickness influences vascular reliability. Lateral and medial approaches show vascular advantages over that which can be observed in inferior and superior pedicles in microdissection anatomic studies. The former may, therefore, be regarded as more reliable.[24] Pedicles other than the inferior pedicle may also confer an improvement in long-term breast shape, with less bottoming out.[25,26]

There is an overall trend toward limited scar techniques and also the use of liposuction as an adjunctive tool, or as the sole means for a smaller reduction. The risk and complication profiles of these are highly surgeon, experience, and patient dependent.[27,28]

AVOIDANCE OF HEMATOMA

Any operative procedure to some degree carries the risk of hematoma. Evidence suggests that intraoperative hypotension in the middle period of the operation, which is usually the period when homeostasis is achieved, is associated with the development of postoperative wound hematoma.[29,30] Avoidance of hematoma is therefore likely best achieved by adequate perioperative control of any preexisting hypertension, ensuring normotensive conditions when obtaining hemostasis (as well as using adjunctive techniques such as temporary Valsalva to identify areas of bleeding) and ensuring an optimal wake up from anesthesia without spikes in blood pressure. Drains do not prevent hematoma and the trend has been away from using closed suction drainage in reduction mammaplasty altogether.[31,32] When hematoma does occur, incision and drainage should be performed given the risk of hematoma-induced tissue necrosis and resultant infectious complications.[33] This may be accomplished by a return to the operating room with reopening the incisions, evacuation of the hematoma, and control of a bleeding point if found versus ultrasound-guided aspiration in selected cases. Suction aspiration can be used for smaller hematomas that have already liquefied—normally 10 to 14 days after surgery.

AVOIDANCE OF SKIN ISCHEMIA, SKIN LOSS, AND WOUND SEPARATION

Some degree of wound separation is very common after breast reduction, as previously stated. Smoking cessation, abstinence from steroid therapy, and control of diabetes or connective tissue diseases are vital. Technical considerations must also be made for the avoidance of skin ischemia that results in skin loss and delayed healing. Enough tissue must be resected from the pedicle such that the wounds are approximated without excess tension. When using the Wise pattern, the point of maximal tension is at the T junction. This pattern of flap closure involves the development of skin flaps and draping of these around a centrally positioned pedicle. For this reason, the sum of the measured lengths of the medial and lateral skin flaps is always longer than the length of the inframammary incision. The lateral flap tends to have a longer length to width ratio with blood supply further from the distal edge than from the edge of the medial flap. Therefore, the lateral flap is more prone to ischemia. It is the authors' belief that skin closure does not contribute significantly to breast shape. Rather, the pedicle must fit the wound created by the flap dissection precisely. Therefore, if there is excessive tension on the closure, resection of additional parenchymal tissue is needed.

AVOIDANCE OF NIPPLE–AREOLA COMPLEX ISCHEMIA

NAC ischemia is among the most dreaded and devastating complications of breast reduction. It occurs owing to arterial insufficiency after resection of breast parenchyma that disrupts NAC perfusion. The authors believe that in secondary breast reduction knowledge of the previous pedicle orientation is crucial. If the previous pedicle is not known, then a resection and nipple transplantation technique is the safest approach for minimizing the risk of nipple loss. Venous insufficiency can occur also if a pedicle is folded excessively during closure. Risk factors for NAC ischemia are a long pedicle (>15 cm from nipple to IMF in an inferior pedicle reduction), nipple transposition distance of greater than 18 cm, and decreases of greater than 2000 g.[1] In these circumstances, an amputation-type reduction with free nipple grafting should be considered. NAC ischemia can occur outside of these parameters and as such all patients should be informed of the possibility of this complication when consenting to undergo reduction mammaplasty. Similarly, focal devascularization can lead to fat necrosis and calcification, which is difficult to predict and also should be discussed as part of an informed consent. Furthermore, monitoring of the NAC viability should be performed throughout the operative procedure. Detection of NAC ischemia intraoperatively can be difficult, especially in dark-skinned patients. As well as checking capillary refill and bleeding skin edges, intravenous fluorescein or using indocyanine green–based perfusion assessment systems can be helpful. When there is concern for NAC viability compromise, the pedicle should be checked for any kinks and vasospasm should be addressed with warm sponges or pharmaceutically, for example, with papavarine. A truly ischemic NAC should be converted to a full-thickness skin graft and inset to a well-vascularized portion of the pedicle or placed on the breast skin after closure.

AVOIDANCE OF UNATTRACTIVE SCARS

As stated, breast reduction represents a "trade-off of size and shape for scars" and preoperative counseling that the scars will be permanent is mandatory. In addition, it is generally accepted that scar tissue healing is not completely predictable in any setting and this independent of who makes the incision and who closes the resulting wound(s). Nonetheless, the surgeon can take certain measures to avoid scars being more unattractive than needs be. Widened and hypertrophic scars can result from closure under significant tension. As described, parenchymal resection must be such to avoid undue tension on the suture line. An extended lateral closure in a bid to shape the breast should be avoided because this only guarantees a worse scar. Dog ears greater than 1 cm should be excised at the time of surgery because they will likely not resolve.

Traditionally, scar treatment strategies have been dominated by cosmeceutical company pseudoscience and marketing, anecdotal evidence, and subjective observations rather than large-scale randomized controlled trials, objective data, and evidence-based techniques. There is no single, optimal topical modality that can eliminate or prevent cutaneous scars be they immature, maturing, mature, hypertrophic, or keloid. Many surgeons have adopted the "low-tech–low-cost" approach of applying adhesive microporous hypoallergenic paper tape applied to fresh surgical incisions, and replaced every 3 to 7 days for up to 12 weeks is useful in low-risk patients to improve scar cosmesis and prevent hypertrophic scarring.[34,35] Silicone gel sheeting is the most accepted modality in the treatment and prevention of hypertrophic scar in high-risk patients (ie, those who have previously suffered abnormal scarring). Use of silicone gel sheeting should begin soon after surgical closure, when the incision has fully epithelialized and be continued for at least 1 month. Silicone gel sheets should be worn for a minimum of 12 hours daily, and if possible for 24 hours per day with twice daily washing.[34] Topical vitamin E, cocoa butter, onion extract cream (eg, Mederma), alantoin-sulfomucopolysaccharide gel, glycosaminoglycan gel, and creams containing extracts form plants such as *Bulbine frutescens* and *Centella astiatica* have not been shown to consistently improve scar appearance as single agents. Any benefits of such topical agents have been suggested to result from massage associated with their application, and as such deep wound massage therapy is a common modality in the management of scarring, although the scientific evidence for its efficacy is also limited.[34,36–38]

AVOIDANCE OF VOLUME AND NIPPLE–AREOLA COMPLEX ASYMMETRY

No 2 breasts are identical, and identification of preexisting asymmetries is essential in avoiding increased or worse asymmetries after breast reduction surgery. All patients should expect some degree of subtle asymmetry and indeed asymmetry may be more apparent on a smaller postreduction breast. Significant preexisting breast volume asymmetry or asymmetry of NAC size, shape, or position requires appropriate operatively planning to design tissue resection and skin incisions accordingly to improve harmony. In the absence of gross preexisting asymmetry, the best practice is to simply "do the same thing to both sides." This may not be as easy as it seems, especially if independent surgeons are working concomitantly on their respective sides as is commonplace. To achieve the best possible symmetry, a patient can be placed in a sitting position at 90° on the operating table so that the breasts can and should be carefully analyzed from the foot of the table. If adjustments in volume, contour, nipple position, or skin envelope draping are necessary, these can be pursued before completion of wound closure.

AVOIDANCE OF NIPPLE–AREOLA COMPLEX MALPOSITION

NAC malposition, typically superior malposition, after reduction mammaplasty is the result of a nipple placed too high at the time of surgery. The NAC does not move, although the volume of breast tissue settles inferiorly with time such that the distance from NAC to IMF increases and the nipple seems to be displaced superiorly. This can be avoided by correct positioning of the NAC in the first place and simply not placing it too high. The authors' preferred technique is to transpose the IMF anteriorly onto the breast to identify the correct level for nipple placement. Placing the nipple slightly lower than the IMF when the residual breast volume is large may be a helpful strategy to minimize the occurrence of "high riding" nipples.

AVOIDANCE OF NIPPLE RETRACTION

Nipple retraction is the result of overresection of breast parenchyma beneath the nipple such that remaining breast parenchymal tissue is inadequate to support the nipple as the most anteriorly projecting aspect of the breast. This is a technical error that can be avoided. Avoidance of this problem is achieved by careful effort to maintain adequate parenchymal tissue in this region at the time of resection by "beveling" the resection away from the NAC in all directions to preserve tissue to support the NAC which should "sit" at or slightly above skin level without the influence of sutures.

SUMMARY

Breast reduction results in smaller, shapelier, more youthful appearing breasts with patients relieved of the symptoms of macromastia in exchange for the "trade-off of scars for symptom improvement and shape." Although numerous complications can occur after reduction mammaplasty, it has been our experience that major complications or those that require surgical revision are exceedingly rare. Outcome studies have repeatedly championed breast reduction and documented high levels of patient satisfaction. Nonetheless, informed consent of risks and possible complications is an important part of preoperatively educating and preparing each patient for surgery and managing patient expectations.

REFERENCES

1. Shestak KC. Re-operative plastic surgery of the breast. Philadelphia: Lippincott Williams & Wilkins; 2006.

2. Cunningham BL, Gear AJ, Kerrigan CL, et al. Analysis of breast reduction complications derived from the BRAVO study. Plast Reconstr Surg 2005; 115(6):1597–604.

3. Strombeck JO. Macromastia in women and its surgical treatment. Acta Chir Scand Suppl 1964;341:84.

4. Dabbah A, Lehman JA Jr, Parker MG, et al. Reduction mammaplasty: an outcome analysis. Ann Plast Surg 1995;35:337.

5. Menke H, Eisenmann-Klein M, Olbrisch RR, et al. Continuous quality management of breast hypertrophy by the German Association of Plastic Surgeons: a preliminary report. Ann Plast Surg 2001;46:594.

6. Zubowski R, Zins JE, Foray-Kaplon A, et al. Relationship of obesity and specimen weight to complications in reduction mammaplasty. Plast Reconstr Surg 2000;106:998.

7. Economides NG, Sifakis F. Reduction mammaplasty: a study of sequelae. Breast J 1997;3:69.

8. Lejour M. Vertical mammaplasty: early complications after 250 personal consecutive cases. Plast Reconstr Surg 1999;104:764.

9. Mandrekas AD, Zambacos GJ, Anastasopoulos A, et al. Reduction mammaplasty with the inferior pedicle technique: early and late complications in 371 patients. Br J Plast Surg 1996;49:442.

10. Setälä L, Papp A, Joukainen S, et al. Obesity and complications in breast reduction surgery: are restrictions justified? J Plast Reconstr Aesthet Surg 2009;62(2):195–9.

11. Roehl K, Craig ES, Gómez V, et al. Breast reduction: safe in the morbidly obese? Plast Reconstr Surg 2008;122(2):370–8.

12. Schumacher HH. Breast reduction and smoking. Ann Plast Surg 2005;54(2):117–9.

13. Bikhchandani J, Varma SK, Henderson HP. Is it justified to refuse breast reduction to smokers? J Plast Reconstr Aesthet Surg 2007;60(9):1050–4.

14. Bartsch RH, Weiss G, Kästenbauer T, et al. Crucial aspects of smoking in wound healing after breast reduction surgery. J Plast Reconstr Aesthet Surg 2007;60(9):1045–9.

15. Krueger JK, Rohrich RJ. Clearing the smoke: the scientific rationale for tobacco abstention with plastic surgery. Plast Reconstr Surg 2001;108(4):1063–73.

16. Rohrich RJ, Coberly DM, Krueger JK, et al. Planning elective operations on patients who smoke: survey of North American plastic surgeons. Plast Reconstr Surg 2002;109(1):350–5.

17. Souto GC, Giugliani ER, Giugliani C, et al. The impact of breast reduction surgery on breastfeeding performance. J Hum Lact 2003;19(1):43–9.

18. Marshall D, Callan P, Nicholson W. Breastfeeding after reduction mammaplasty. Br J Plast Surg 1994; 47(3):167–9.

19. Harris L, Morris SF, Freiberg A. Is breast feeding possible after reduction mammaplasty? Plast Reconstr Surg 1992;89(5):836–9.

20. Brzozowski D, Niessen M, Evans HB, et al. Breastfeeding after inferior pedicle reduction mammaplasty. Plast Reconstr Surg 2000;105(2):530–4.

21. Colwell AS, Kukreja J, Breuing KH, et al. Occult breast carcinoma in reduction mammaplasty specimens: 14-year experience. Plast Reconstr Surg 2004;113(7):1984–8.

22. Scott GR, Carson CL, Borah GL. Maximizing outcomes in breast reduction surgery: a review of 518 consecutive patients. Plast Reconstr Surg 2005; 116(6):1633–9.

23. Jackson IT, Bayramicli M, Gupta M, et al. Importance of the pedicle length measurement in reduction mammaplasty. Plast Reconstr Surg 1999;104(2):398–400.

24. Cruz-Korchin N, Korchin L. Vertical versus wise pattern breast reduction: patient satisfaction, revision rates, and complications. Plast Reconstr Surg 2003;112(6):1573–8.

25. mon O'Dey D, Prescher A, Pallua N. Vascular reliability of nipple-areola complex–bearing pedicles: an anatomical microdissection study. Plast Reconstr Surg 2007;119(4):1167–77.

26. Abramson DL, Pap S, Shifteh S, et al. Improving long-term breast shape with the medial pedicle wise pattern breast reduction. Plast Reconstr Surg 2005;115(7):1937–43.

27. Strauch B, Elkowitz M, Baum T, et al. Superolateral pedicle for breast surgery: an operation for all reasons. Plast Reconstr Surg 2005;115(5):1269–77.

28. Rohrich RJ, Gosman AA, Brown SA, et al. Current preferences for breast reduction techniques: a survey of board-certified plastic surgeons 2002. Plast Reconstr Surg 2004;114(7):1724–33.

29. Okoro SA, Barone C, Bohnenblust M, et al. Breast reduction trend among plastic surgeons: a national survey. Plast Reconstr Surg 2008;122(5):1312–20.

30. Hussien M, Lee S, Webster M, et al. The impact of intraoperative hypotension on the development of wound haematoma after breast reduction. Br J Plast Surg 2001;54(6):517–22.

31. Henry SL, Crawford JL, Puckett CL. Risk factors and complications in reduction mammaplasty: novel associations and preoperative assessment. Plast Reconstr Surg 2009;124(4):1040–6.

32. Collis N, McGuiness CM, Batchelor AG. Drainage in breast reduction surgery: a prospective randomised intra-patient trail. Br J Plast Surg 2005; 58(3):286–9.

33. Wrye SW, Banducci DR, Mackay D, et al. Routine drainage is not required in reduction mammaplasty. Plast Reconstr Surg 2003;111(1):113–7.

34. Angel MF, Narayanan K, Swartz WM, et al. The etiologic role of free radicals in hematoma-induced flap necrosis. Plast Reconstr Surg 1986;77(5):795–801.

35. Mustoe TA, Cooter RD, Gold MH, et al. International clinical recommendations on scar management. Plast Reconstr Surg 2002;110:560–71.

36. Reiffel RS. Prevention of hypertrophic scars by long-term paper tape application. Plast Reconstr Surg 1995;96(7):1715–8.

37. Foo CW, Tristani-Firouzi P. Topical modalities for treatment and prevention of postsurgical hypertrophic scars. Facial Plast Surg Clin North Am 2011; 19(3):551–7.

38. Havlik RJ. Vitamin E and wound healing: safety and efficacy reports. Plast Reconstr Surg 1997;100:1901–2.

Reduction Mammaplasty and Breast Cancer Screening

Yan T. Ortiz-Pomales, MD[a], Priyanka Handa, MD[b],
Mary S. Newell, MD[b], Albert Losken, MD[a],*

KEYWORDS

- Breast reduction • Reduction mammaplasty • Cancer screening • Imaging findings • Mammogram

KEY POINTS

- There are no evidence-based data to confirm the utility of unique screening protocols for women undergoing reduction mammaplasty surgery.
- Postoperative screening mammography does not lead to significantly more imaging or diagnostic interventions when compared with nonoperative controls.
- Parenchymal redistribution occurs in 90% of cases and can be seen at mammography and MRI.
- Fat necrosis is common after breast reduction and usually has an easily identifiable appearance on mammography. In its mature form, it can be seen as an oil cyst, which is a lucent, fat-density round or oval mass on mammogram, often with classic rim calcifications at its periphery.
- MRI and ultrasound features of the postreduction mammaplasty breast parallel some of the mammographic findings commonly seen in mammography.

INTRODUCTION

Breast reduction surgery is a safe and popular cosmetic procedure for the treatment of symptoms associated with breast hypertrophy. According to the Cosmetic Surgery National Data Bank published in 2014, a total of 114,170 breast reductions were performed in the United States last year; it currently ranks as the eighth most common cosmetic surgery done in this country.[1]

This surgery's great popularity is due to its success in treating both the complex psychological and physical sequela associated with this disease process.[2] Although generally this procedure has high patient satisfaction,[3] patients are often concerned about this surgery's impact on the diagnostic accuracy of postprocedural mammography for routine cancer screenings.

The indications for this particular surgery are clear and defined as a syndrome of persistent

Disclaimers: The views expressed in this article are those of the authors and do not necessarily reflect the official policy or position of the Department of the Navy, Department of Defense, or the US government.
Dr Y.O.-P. is a military service member (or employee of the US government). This work was prepared as part of his official duties. Title 17, USC, §105 provides that "Copyright protection under this title is not available for any work of the U.S. Government." Title 17, USC, §101 defines a US government work as a work prepared by a military service member or employee of the US government as part of that person's official duties.
[a] Division of Plastic and Reconstructive Surgery, Emory University, 550 Peachtree Street, Suite 84300, Atlanta, GA 30308, USA; [b] Division of Plastics and Reconstructive Surgery, Department of Radiology, Emory University, 550 Peachtree Street, Suite 84300, Atlanta, GA 30308, USA
* Corresponding author.
E-mail address: alosken@emory.edu

Clin Plastic Surg 43 (2016) 333–339
http://dx.doi.org/10.1016/j.cps.2015.12.009
0094-1298/16/$ – see front matter © 2016 Elsevier Inc. All rights reserved.

plasticsurgery.theclinics.com

neck and shoulder pain, painful shoulder grooving from brassiere straps, and chronic intertriginous rash of the inframammary fold caused by an increase in the volume and weight of breast tissue beyond normal proportions. Breast hypertrophy can be associated with significant fibrous breast parenchyma and increased breast density that already poses a decrease in mammogram sensitivity and specificity as a screening method for malignancy.

Although women undergoing reduction mammaplasty are expected to continue routine radiologic screenings for breast cancer, significant debate exists about the current recommendations for screening in the general population. This lack of clear consensus affects our preoperative counseling to patients seeking reduction mammaplasty.[4,5]

In this article, the authors review the current recommendations for cancer screening with mammography, common radiologic findings after mammaplasty that may impact false-positive tests leading to increase call back numbers. The authors also examine the impact of postsurgical radiographic changes on recognizing breast cancer in this population.

Preoperative Screening Recommendations

There are no evidence-based data to confirm the utility of unique screening protocols for women undergoing reduction mammaplasty surgery or for those who already have had reduction. For average-risk women in general, annual screening mammography for women 40 years of age and older is recommended by the American Cancer Society, the American College of Surgeons, The American College of Radiology, and the American Congress of Obstetricians and Gynecologists. Among women younger than 40 years, the evidence supports screening mammography only for those who have a high risk for breast cancer.[6] There is a logical appeal to obtaining a presurgical baseline mammogram in patients younger than 40 years to diminish the likelihood of an unanticipated occult cancer being found on pathologic examination of the excised breast tissue. However, the incidence of cancer in this age group is low; there are no robust data to support the efficacy of this approach. It is imperative, of course, for the surgeon to identify concerning aspects of the patients' history or findings on physical examination in the preoperative setting that would suggest the need for further investigation with diagnostic, rather than screening, imaging evaluation.

IMAGING FINDINGS POSTREDUCTION MAMMAPLASTY

Regardless of the exact type of reduction procedure performed, the changes seen on imaging reflect the removal and repositioning of breast tissue and the nipple-areolar complex and any associated resultant scarring.[7] Although the traditional inverted-T scar, or Wise pattern, involves both an inframammary fold incision and a vertical incision, newer vertical scar techniques feature a vertical incision alone. The use of the vertical incision decreases scarring and distortion of the inframammary fold, and it aids in shaping the breast by allowing various techniques for parenchymal rearrangement and pedicle creation.[8]

For the surgically altered breast, some investigators suggest obtaining a mammogram 6 to 12 months after surgery to reestablish baseline findings.[9] However, when compared with a control group of patients who did not undergo surgery, patients who underwent reduction mammaplasty did not have a significant difference in mammographic abnormalities (defined as a Breast Imaging Reporting and Data System category 3, 4, or 5 lesions).[9] Breast reduction mammaplasty changes do not decrease the specificity of the screening mammograms as there was no difference in the rate of recall for women for further assessment. Therefore, the practice of obtaining mammographic imaging outside of routine screening intervals is likely not medically necessary or warranted. Despite the substantial tissue mobilization performed during reduction mammaplasty, postoperative screening mammography does not lead to significantly more imaging or diagnostic interventions when compared with nonoperative controls.[10,11] Interestingly, these investigators noted a decreased rate of breast cancer in the breast-reduction group, which is in keeping with previous study findings.[11]

MAMMOGRAPHY

The common mammographic findings associated with reduction surgery include alteration of breast contour, elevation of the nipple, displacement of breast parenchyma, architectural distortion, skin thickening, fibrotic bands of scar, and fat necrosis.

Parenchymal redistribution occurs in 90% of cases and can be seen at mammography and MRI (**Fig. 1**).[12] The inverted-T horizontal skin incision is seen at imaging as dermal calcifications, skin thickening, or keloids along the inframammary

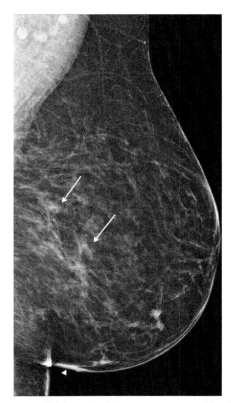

Fig. 1. Medial lateral oblique mammographic view shows a band of mildly distorted tissue (*long arrows*) obliquely oriented in breast, unusual in distribution for normal breast parenchyma but typical for postreduction change. Note skin thickening in inframammary fold region (*arrowhead*), also a common in postreduction change.

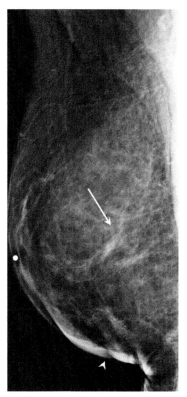

Fig. 2. Medial lateral oblique view in another patient, showing the characteristic postreduction band of scar tissue (*long arrow*) and significant skin thickening (*arrowhead*) extending from nipple inferiorly to inframammary fold. Note how high the nipple is situated on the breast, marker by metallic BB.

fold. Placement of scar markers on the skin surface may be helpful to localize these findings as lying within the dermis. Vertically oriented skin thickening related to the vertical skin incision can also be seen at imaging (**Fig. 2**).[13]

Architectural distortion (**Fig. 3**) may be seen after any type of breast surgery, including reduction. In most cases, its cause is clear-cut; but salient history of the prior surgery and knowledge of the typical postreduction pattern is extremely helpful, as on occasion, cancers can present as isolated distortions. On occasion, patients may be recalled for further evaluation of architectural distortion seen during the course of routine screening after prior reduction. If the finding cannot be definitely dismissed as postsurgical, needle biopsy may be required to exclude neoplasm, as all distortions cannot be presumed postsurgical benign, especially if new or progressing.

Fat necrosis is common after breast reduction and usually has an easily identifiable appearance on mammography but can present a diagnostic dilemma on occasion. In its mature form, it can be seen as an oil cyst, which is a lucent, fat-density round or oval mass on mammogram, often with classic rim calcifications at its periphery (**Fig. 4**). However, earlier in its evolution, fat necrosis may present as patchy soft tissue density, distortion, or even a discrete mass that is indistinguishable from breast cancer (**Figs. 5** and **6**). Along the same lines, the calcifications often seen with fat necrosis may sometimes seem suspicious. They tend to become coarser and more dystrophic over time; but when they first appear mammographically, they can resemble fine pleomorphic calcifications that can be seen associated with ductal carcinoma in situ (DCIS) or invasive ductal cancers (**Fig. 7**).

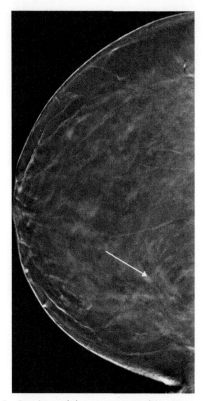

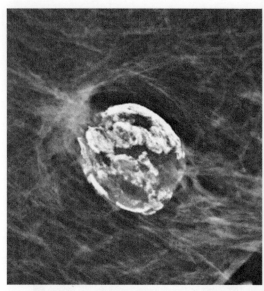

Fig. 4. Classic benign appearance of an oil cyst, commonly seen in the setting of prior breast reduction. Note the lucent center and rim calcifications. No additional evaluation is required, even if it is palpable, as this finding was.

Fig. 3. Craniocaudal mammographic image performed with digital breast tomosynthesis, accounting for its blurred appearance, except for the architectural distortion (*long arrow*), which is in focus on this tomographic slice. Knowing postreduction history and confirming imaging stability helps indicate its benign nature in this case, as distortions like this can represent breast cancer.

ULTRASOUND AND MRI

MRI and ultrasound features of the postreduction mammaplasty breast parallel some of the mammographic findings discussed earlier. Findings that may be discernable on these modalities include parenchymal redistribution, fat necrosis, and scarring (**Fig. 8**).

Sagittal T1-weighted sequences after reduction mammaplasty best demonstrate a predominance of breast parenchymal tissue in the inferior dependent portion of the breast. Parenchymal redistribution is seen postoperatively because of resection of the subcutaneous fat.[12] Ultrasound cannot detect tissue redistribution.

Fat necrosis is commonly seen in the inferior, central breast after reduction mammaplasty.[14] On ultrasound, fat necrosis is variable in appearance ranging from ill-defined to circumscribed masses with mixed internal echotexture (**Fig. 9**). It can on occasion present as a solid mass with internal vascular flow, which may necessitate biopsy. However, if the finding can be seen to lie in region of the surgical bed, close follow-up may be pursued rather than biopsy.

As fat necrosis typically follows fat signal on magnetic resonance sequences, it usually can be differentiated from malignancy despite the fact that it often demonstrates robust contrast enhancement, especially when an inflammatory component is present.[15] The most common MRI appearance of fat necrosis is that of a lipid cyst with or without a fat-fluid level. A round or oval mass with hypointense T1-weighted signal on fat-saturated images is typical. It may show black-fat appearance on T1- and T2-weighted images, with its central contents appearing even darker than adjacent viable fat signal. The rim of an oil cyst/area of fat necrosis commonly enhance, although to varying degrees. On occasion, the lack of clear-cut internal fat signal, combined with enhancement, may necessitate correlative imaging with mammography or ultrasound. Rarely, if corresponding pathognomonic finding of fat necrosis are not found, needle biopsy or short-interval follow-up may be required for clarification.

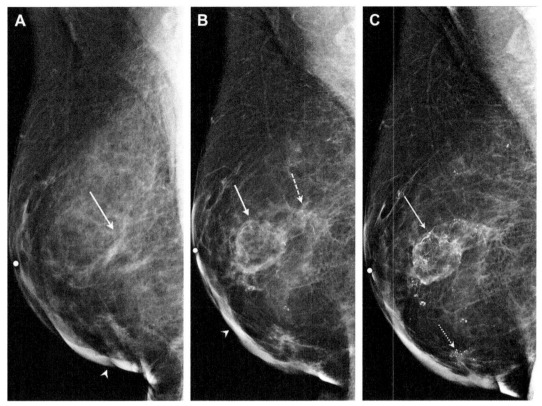

Fig. 5. Mammographic evolution of fat necrosis. (*A*) One year after surgery, minor findings are seen, showing the characteristic postreduction band of scar tissue (*long arrow*) and significant skin thickening (*arrowhead*) extending from nipple inferiorly to inframammary fold. (*B*) One year later, an oil cyst with early calcifications (*solid arrow*) and patchy scar tissue (*dashed arrow*) are forming. Skin thickening (*arrowhead*) persists. (*C*). Three years after the procedure, the oil cyst is maturing with coarsening calcifications at it rim (*solid arrow*). An emerging architectural distortion is seen inferiorly (*dashed arrow*), a finding that may require added evaluation but in this case proved to be scar.

Enhancement of the inframammary fold and skin and a focus of susceptibility artifact are compatible with hypertrophic scarring (keloids) from reduction mammaplasty.[12] Ultrasound is not typically helpful in the setting of postsurgical scarring as it presents with a hypoechoic mass with posterior shadowing mimicking malignancy.[15] A linear hypoechoic line extending from the area of shadowing to the skin surface can be useful in distinguishing scar from malignancy. Imaging of postsurgical scars on MRI varies depending on the timeline. In most cases, enhancement within the biopsy bed is seen up to 12 months after surgery.[15]

FOLLOWING ONCOPLASTIC BREAST REDUCTION

In a study at the authors' institution, they demonstrated that following partial breast reconstruction using reduction techniques mammography was just as sensitive as a screening tool when compared with patients with breast conservation therapy (BCT) alone.[16] Although the qualitative mammographic findings were similar in the two groups over the average 6-year follow-up, there was a slight trend toward longer times to mammographic stability in the oncoplastic reduction group (25.6 months vs 21.2 months in the BCT alone group). This finding means it might take the oncoplastic reduction patients slightly longer to reach the point where any change in mammographic findings might be suspicious for malignancy. There was a higher rate of tissue sampling in the reduction group (53% vs 18%, $P = .015$). The clinical significance of this finding remains to be seen. An accurate interpretation of mammography requires familiarity with these temporal changes, and mammograms should be compared over time. These data need to be taken into consideration when designing the most appropriate surveillance programs for these patients.

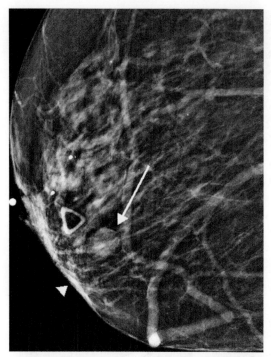

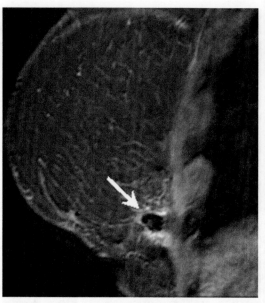

Fig. 8. Postcontrast T1-weighted sagittal MRI shows fat necrosis in a typical postreduction location in inferior breast (*arrow*). Note their irregular enhancement, which can also be seen in cancer. However, the central black fat confirms the cause as fat necrosis.

Fig. 6. Subcentimeter circumscribed oval mass is seen at the site of a palpable lump (location outlined by a radio-opaque triangle marker placed on the skin by the technologist) in this postreduction patient (*long arrow*). This finding is nonspecific and can be seen with fat necrosis. However, as it was new, ultrasound correlation was required (see **Fig. 7**) to exclude malignancy (*Arrowhead* shows the significant skin thickening).

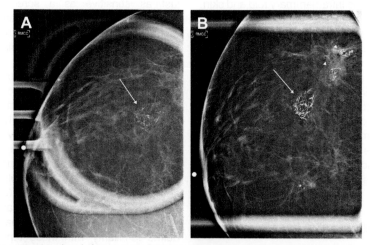

Fig. 7. Calcifications associated with fat necrosis. (*A*) First postreduction mammogram shows grouped fine pleomorphic calcifications arranged in an area of lucent tissue (*long arrow*). Although these are intrinsically suspicious in appearance, the presence of intervening fat (lucency) and knowledge of the recent surgery type allow these to be assessed as very likely related to evolving fat necrosis rather than DCIS and followed rather than subjected to biopsy. (*B*) Follow-up mammogram 6 months later shows that the calcifications have coarsened, typical now of fat necrosis (*long arrow*). Note other areas of evolving fat necrosis with distortion, central lucency, and calcifications (*arrowheads*).

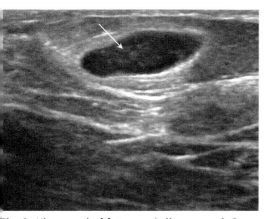

Fig. 9. Ultrasound of fat necrosis (*long arrow*). Sonographic evaluation of the mass seen in **Fig. 6** shows a complex cystic and solid mass. Note the internal echogenicity, precluding dismissal as a simple cyst. However, its avascular nature on color Doppler images (*not shown*) and knowledge of surgical history suggest fat necrosis as the cause.

SUMMARY

Breast reduction surgery is one of the most popular procedures performed by plastic surgeons; based on the current literature, it is safe and does not have any negative impact on identifying breast cancer in women. It is important to highlight that there are no evidence-based data to confirm the utility of unique screening protocols for women planning to undergo reduction surgery or for those who already have had reduction. Women undergoing this surgery should not deviate from the current recommendations of screening mammography in women older than 40 years of average risk. Although tempting, there are not enough date to support the use of routine baseline mammogram before breast reduction, as the risk of occult disease is extremely low. It is up to the surgeon to preoperatively identify any reason to obtain the appropriate studies on patients at high risk before proceeding with any elective breast surgery.

REFERENCES

1. ASPS Cosmetic Surgery National Data Bank Statistics 2014.
2. Glatt B, Sarwer D, O'Hara D, et al. A retrospective study of changes in physical symptoms and body image after reduction mammaplasty. Plast Reconstr Surg 1999;103:76.
3. Davis GM, Ringler S, Short K, et al. Reduction mammaplasty: long-term efficacy, morbidity, and patient satisfaction. Plast Reconstr Surg 1995;96(5):1106–10.
4. Meissner HI, Rimer BK, Davis WW, et al. Another round in the mammography controversy. J Womens Health (Larchmt) 2003;12:261–76.
5. Fletcher SW. Why question screening mammography for women in their forties? Radiol Clin North Am 1995;33:1259–71.
6. Kerrigan CL, Slezak SS. Evidence-based medicine: reduction mammaplasty. Plast Reconstr Surg 2013;132:1670.
7. Bassett LW, Mahoney MC, Apple SK, et al. Breast imaging. The surgically altered breast: breast imaging. 1st edition. Philadelphia: Saunders; 2011. p. 682–9.
8. Hamdi M, Hammond DC, Nahai F. Vertical scar mammaplasty. Heidelberg (Germany): Springer; 2005.
9. Thongchai P. The surgically altered breast: imaging technique and findings. Gland Surg 2014;3:48–50.
10. Roberts JM, Clark CJ, Campbell MJ, et al. Incidence of abnormal mammograms after reduction mammoplasty: implications for oncoplastic closure. Am J Surg 2011;201:611–4.
11. Muir TM, Tresham J, Fritschi L, et al. Screening for breast cancer post reduction mammoplasty. Clin Radiol 2010;65:198–205.
12. Margolis NE, Christopher Morley C, Philip Lotfi P, et al. Update on imaging of the post-surgical breast. Radiographics 2014;34:642–60.
13. Danikas D, Theodorou SJ, Kokkalis G, et al. Mammographic findings following reduction mammoplasty. Aesthetic Plast Surg 2001;25:283–5.
14. Daly CP, Jaeger B, Sill DS. Variable appearances of fat necrosis on breast MRI. AJR Am J Roentgenol 2008;191:1374–80.
15. Shaheen R, Schimmelpenninck CA, Stoddart L, et al. Spectrum of diseases presenting as architectural distortion on mammography: multimodality radiologic imaging with pathologic correlation. Semin Ultrasound CT MR 2011;32:351–62.
16. Losken A, Schaefer TG, Newell M, et al. The impact of partial breast reconstruction using reduction techniques on post-operative cancer surveillance. Plast Reconstr Surg 2009;124(1):9–17.

The Management of Breast Cancer Detected by Reduction Mammaplasty

Grant W. Carlson, MD

KEYWORDS

• Reduction mammaplasty • Occult cancer • Contralateral symmetry

KEY POINTS

• Occult breast cancer detected by reduction mammaplasty is 0.06% to 5.45%; The incidence is higher in older women and if the reduction is performed as a symmetry procedure for contralateral breast cancer.
• Preoperative screening mammography is indicated in all women 40 years and older and in women age 35 with a positive family or personal history before reduction mammaplasty.
• Two-thirds of cases found at the time of reduction mammaplasty are noninvasive and the majority are mammographically occult.
• Management of occult cancer is impacted by specimens being removed in pieces and not oriented before submission to pathology. Total mastectomy is common because of uncertainties regarding margin status and disease extent.

INTRODUCTION

Reduction mammaplasty is one of the most commonly performed plastic surgery procedures. The American Society of Plastic Surgeons estimates 110,000 women in the United States underwent reduction mammaplasty for symptomatic macromastia or for symmetry in 2014.[1,2] The incidence of occult cancer detected after breast reduction mammaplasties is very low, ranging from 0.06% to 5.45%[3-7] (**Table 1**). The incidence is higher in older women and if the reduction is performed as a symmetry procedure for a patient with a history of contralateral cancer.[8-11] Tang and colleagues[7] used the Ontario Cancer Registry to examine the incidence of invasive breast cancer found at the time of bilateral breast reduction. A total of 27,500 women were studied, 17 (0.06%) were found to have invasive breast cancer. The mean age of women with breast cancer found at the time of breast reduction was 49 years. In comparison, the overall mean age of women in the general population diagnosed with breast cancer was 61 years. Cancers found in the reduction mammaplasty patients were at an earlier

stage and had a better survival than the control group.

FACTORS INFLUENCING THE INCIDENCE OF OCCULT BREAST CANCER FOUND AFTER REDUCTION MAMMAPLASTY
Age

The majority of women undergoing breast reduction for symptomatic macromastia are less than 40 years old (see **Table 1**). Breast cancer is extremely rare in this age group. Clark and colleagues[4] reported the pathologic findings of 562 patients undergoing reduction mammaplasty. They found no atypia or breast cancer in any women younger than age 30. Ambaye and colleagues[3] in their review of 202 women found significant pathologic findings (carcinoma or atypical hyperplasia) in 25 patients (12.4%). Almost all of these findings (23 of 25; 92%) were in women 40 or older.

Family History of Cancer

Thirteen percent of women diagnosed have a first-degree relative (mother, sister, or daughter) with

Department of Surgery, School of Medicine, Emory University, 1365C Clifton Road, Atlanta, GA 30322, USA
E-mail address: gcarlso@emory.edu

Clin Plastic Surg 43 (2016) 341–347
http://dx.doi.org/10.1016/j.cps.2015.12.001
0094-1298/16/$ – see front matter

Table 1
Incidental breast cancer detected after reduction mammaplasty

Study, Year	Patients (n)	Mean Age (y)	History of Breast Cancer	Incidence (per patient)	% Overall Carcinoma (per patient)
Jansen et al,[27] 1998	2576	NS	No	4 (0.16)	0.16
Tang et al,[7] 1999	27,500	49	No	17 (0.06)[b]	0.06
Ishag et al,[6] 2003	518	NS	No	IC: 2 (0.39) DCIS: 1 (0.19)	0.58
Ishag et al,[6] 2003	42	NS	Yes	IC: 1 (2.4)	2.38
Colwell et al,[8] 2004	611	38	No	IC: 2 (0.3) DCIS: 2 (0.3)	0.07
Colwell et al,[8] 2004	170	61	Yes	IC: 1 (0.6) DCIS 1 (0.6)	1.18
Cook et al,[5] 2004	1289	36.8	—	IC: 1 (0.1) DCIS: 4 (0.3)	0.31
Dotto et al,[21] 2008	516	35	No	IC: 1 (0.19) DCIS: 1 (0.19)	0.39
Ambaye et al,[3,c] 2009	181	NS	No	IC: 2 (1.1) DCIS: 3 (1.7)	2.76
Clark et al,[4] 2009	562	[a]	NS	DCIS: 6 (1.1)	1.1
Slezak et al,[22] 2011	629	NS	No	IC: 3 DCIS: 6	0.95
Hassan et al,[9] 2012	1061	37	No	IC: 1 (0.09) DCIS: 4 (0.38)	0.05
Hassan et al,[9] 2012	220	52	Yes	IC: 3 (1.36) DCIS: 1 (0.45)	1.82
Desouki et al,[20] 2013	2498	41	No	IC: 2 (0.08) DCIS: 4 (0.16)	0.24
Tadler et al,[11] 2014	479	NS	No	DCIS: 2 (0.42)	0.42
Tadler et al,[11] 2014	55	NS	Yes	DCIS: 3 (5.45)	5.45
Sorin et al,[10] 2015	2718	54.0	Yes	IC: 12 (0.44) DCIS: 28 (1.03)	1.47

Abbreviations: DCIS, ductal carcinoma in situ; IC, invasive cancer; NS, not stated.
[a] Patients with history of breast cancer mean age 52, patients without history of breast cancer mean age 42.
[b] Invasive cancer only.
[c] Increased pathologic sampling.

breast cancer.[12] A woman who has a first-degree relative with breast cancer has almost twice the risk of a woman without a family history. Hereditary breast cancer accounts for 5% to 10% of all cases.[13] It is characterized by having multiple first-degree relatives having had breast cancer, diagnosis at a young age, bilateral breast cancer, and a history of ovarian carcinoma. Inherited gene mutations such as BRCA1 and BRCA2 confer a 45% to 65% risk of developing breast cancer, respectively.

Previous Breast Biopsy Showing High-Risk Pathology

Previous breast biopsies showing atypical ductal hyperplasia, and atypical and lobular carcinoma in situ increases the risk of future breast cancer

development. Atypical pathology confers a moderately increased risk (4–5 times) and LCIS markedly increased risk (8–10 times) of developing breast cancer.[14,15]

Personal History of Breast Cancer

A personal history of breast cancer is a strong risk factor for the development of a new breast cancer. The majority of women with a history of breast cancer take hormonal therapy (tamoxifen, anastrozole, or letrozole), which decreases the risk of new primary cancers by of 50% to 60%. The incidence of occult breast cancer being detected by contralateral breast reduction in women undergoing a symmetry procedure after breast cancer treatment has been reported to be 1.18% to

5.45%[8–11] (see **Table 1**). This is much greater than the incidence of occult cancer found after breast reduction for symptomatic macromastia. Tadler and colleagues[11] found that the prevalence of in situ breast cancer discovered incidentally in reduction mammaplasty specimens was significantly higher for patients with previous history of contralateral breast cancer than for patients without previous breast cancer history (5.5% vs 0.4%; P = .009).

Thoroughness of Preoperative Examination: Imaging

Preoperative mammography is the most practical and cost-effective method for screening of occult malignancy. Despite this, a 2009 national survey in the United Kingdom regarding the use of preoperative mammograms in patients undergoing bilateral reduction mammaplasty revealed a disturbing trend. Whereas 92% of breast surgeons routinely ordered preoperative breast imaging, only 38% of plastic surgeons did so.[16]

Routine screening mammography is recommended by the American Cancer Society to begin at age 40 for the general population. Younger women have denser breasts reducing the sensitivity of screening mammography. This is counterbalanced by the low incidence of cancer in this age group. Slow growing malignancies and low-grade ductal carcinoma in situ without comedo necrosis are more difficult to detect on imaging. Breast MRI scanning is useful in patients with dense breasts, a previous history of breast cancer, and patients with hereditary breast cancer syndromes.

Thoroughness of Postoperative Examination: Pathology

Plastic surgeons routinely submit breast reduction tissue for pathologic evaluation, but there are no standardized procedure for processing and examining these specimens.[5,17,18] Pathologic examination is made more difficult by the often piecemeal removal of breast tissue, which is characteristic of the procedure. After gross evaluation, the number of tissue sections submitted varies by institution. Most ductal carcinoma in situ is not visible of gross examination and less than 1% of all the breast tissue is examined, because total examination would be cost prohibitive.

The Royal College of Pathologist stated that the value of random histology of reduction mammaplasty specimens in patients with symptomatic macromastia is limited.[19] Despite this, microscopic examination of macroscopically normal breast tissue may reveal high-risk pathology, which could alter future breast screening practice.

The risk of finding high-risk lesions (atypical ductal hyperplasia, atypical and lobular carcinoma in situ) in breast reduction specimens for symptomatic macromastia varies from 0.6% and 4.6%.[3,4,8,20–22]

Increased tissue sampling is associated with greater frequency of significant pathologic findings in women older than 40.[3,20] Desouki and colleagues[20] examined the sampling practices of 2 medical centers. One submitted a mean of 7.2 reduction specimens for histology; the other submitted a mean of 3 specimens. The incidence of atypical proliferative lesions detected in the more thorough examinations was 4.6% versus 1.8% (P = .03) in the center that submitted fewer samples.[20] Ambaye and colleagues[3] examined breast reduction specimens with baseline gross and microscopic evaluations as well as additional sampling in 202 women. Increased tissue sampling was associated with significant pathologic findings in women 40 years or older.

MANAGEMENT OF INCIDENTALLY DETECTED BREAST CANCER

Two-thirds of reported cases of breast cancer found incidentally at the time of reduction mammaplasty are noninvasive (**Table 2**). The majority being mammographically occult and only detected by blind tissue sampling. This implies an indolent tumor biology, which may never have become clinically relevant. Invasive cancers tend to be small, the majority being 10 mm or less in diameter. Management of occult cancer is complicated by the fact that specimens are typically removed in pieces and not oriented before submitting them to pathology (**Fig. 1**). Piecemeal removal can make assessment of tumor size difficult. Close or positive margins are problematic because it cannot be determined what represents the true margin. Because of the uncertainties surrounding the extent of disease and margin status in patients with tumors found incidentally during reduction mammaplasty, mastectomy has been the most common treatment.

Specimen orientation is important and could increase the potential for margin reexcision if incidental cancer detected. Sorin and colleagues,[10] in a large multicenter study of 2718 patients, found that only 25% of breast reduction specimens were correctly oriented. Routine orientation should include one marking suture lateral, 2 sutures cranial, and 3 sutures superficial if skin is not included. En bloc resection facilitates pathologic examination. If additional resection is necessary, a suture is positioned on the side of the remaining breast tissue.

Slezak and Bluebond-Langner[22] reported 10 patients who were found to have occult breast

Table 2
Tumor staging of occult cancer after reduction mammaplasty

Study, Year	n	Indication	Cancer, n (%)	DCIS, n (%)	Invasive T1a (%)	T1b (%)	T1c (%)	T2 (%)	NS (%)
Ishag et al,[6] 2003	518	Macromastia	3 (0.58)	1 (33.3)	2 (66.7)	0	0	0	0
Ishag et al,[6] 2003	42	Symmetry	1 (2.4)	0 (0)	0	0	1 (100)	0	0
Colwell et al,[8] 2004	611	Macromastia	4 (0.65)	2 (50)	0	0	2 (50)	0	0
Colwell et al,[8] 2004	170	Symmetry	2 (1.2)	1 (50)	1 (50)	0	0	0	0
Cook et al,[5] 2004	1289	NS	5 (0.39)	4 (80)	0	0	1 (20)	0	0
Dotto et al,[21] 2008	516	Macromastia	2 (0.39)	1 (50)	0	1 (50)	0	0	0
Ambaye et al,[3] 2009	181	Macromastia	5 (2.8)	3 (60)	2 (40)	0	0	0	0
Clark et al,[4] 2009	562	NS	6 (1.1)	6 (100)	0	0	0	0	0
Slezak et al,[22] 2011	629	Macromastia	9 (1.4)	6 (66.7)	1 (11.1)	1 (11.1)	0	1[a] (11.1)	0
Desouki et al,[20] 2013	2498	Macromastia	4 (0.16)	2 (50)	2 (50)	0	0	0	0
Tadler et al,[11] 2014	479	Macromastia	2 (0.42)	2 (100)	0	0	0	0	0
Tadler et al,[11] 2014	55	Symmetry	3 (5.5)	3 (100)	0	0	0	0	0
Sorin et al,[10] 2015	2718	Symmetry	31 (1.1)	19 (61.3)	0	0	0	0	12 (38.7)
Total	10,268	—	77 (0.75)	50 (64.9)	8	2	4	1	12

Total 50/77 (64.9%) DCIS: macromastia 17/29 (58.6%), symmetry 23/36 (63.9%).
   27 cases if interstitial cystitis: T1a 8, T1b 2, T1c 4, T2 1.
   Abbreviations: DCIS, ductal carcinoma in situ; NS, not stated.
   [a] Tubular carcinoma.

cancer after reduction mammaplasty. All the specimens had been routinely oriented. Six were felt to have adequate resection margins and underwent radiation. Two patients had reexcisions, one of whom had persistent margin involvement necessitating total mastectomy.

Breast conservation may be possible if there is a small amount of carcinoma in a limited number of samples. Total mastectomy is the best option if tumor is breast in multiple samples. In cases of small, low-grade, noninvasive or invasive cancer, mastectomy could be delayed for several months.

This time period would allow revascularization of the nipple–areolar complex from the surrounding skin permitting performance of a nipple-sparing mastectomy[23] (**Fig. 2**). Systemic or hormonal therapy could be administered before definitive surgery as determined by gene expression analysis of the tumor.

Sentinel lymph node biopsy is the standard of care for staging breast malignancies. Reduction mammaplasty disrupts the lymphatic pathology, making lymphatic mapping inaccurate in the management of occult breast cancers. Tumor size, hormone receptor analysis, and HER2 overexpression help guide the necessity of axillary lymph node staging.

SUMMARY

1. Thorough history is necessary before reduction mammaplasty to identify any risk factors for breast cancer (personal or family history, high-risk pathology).
2. Preoperative clinical breast examination and counseling regarding the risk and implications of detecting occult breast cancer at the time of reduction mammaplasty are required.
3. Screening mammography before reduction mammaplasty should be performed in all

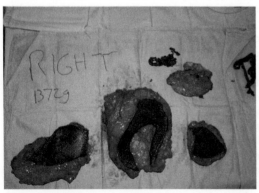

Fig. 1. Intraoperative photograph of inferior pedicle breast reduction specimen.

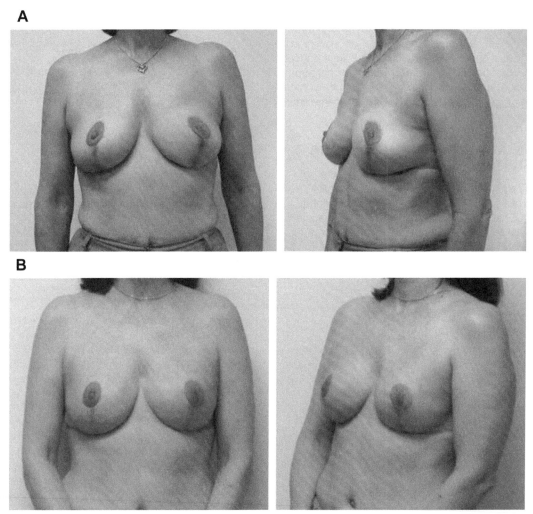

Fig. 2. (*A*) Preoperative photographs: 52-year-old woman status post bilateral superior-medial pedicle breast reduction. Occult lobular carcinoma in situ was detected in random tissue sampling. (*B*) Postoperative photographs: the patient underwent bilateral nipple-sparing mastectomies and immediate reconstruction with 450-mL high-profile breast implants.

women 40 years and older and in women age 35 with a positive family or personal history of breast cancer. Breast MRI is considered in women with dense breasts and those with hereditary breast cancer syndromes.

4. Pathologic analysis of reduction mammaplasty specimens should include patients with a previous history of breast cancer, patients 30 years and older, and patients with a significant family history of breast cancer or those with a hereditary breast cancer syndrome.

5. Routine orientation of breast reduction specimens and en bloc resection should be performed if possible, especially in women with personal or family history of breast cancer.

6. The treatment of the occult breast cancers depends on several factors, including:

a. Previous breast cancer history,
b. Surgical margin evaluation, and
c. Family history.

REDUCTION MAMMAPLASTY AND THE RISK OF BREAST CANCER

Retrospective studies suggest that removal of breast tissue correlates with a reduced risk of breast cancer. Tarone and colleagues[24] performed a review of 6 epidemiologic studies of breast cancer after reduction mammaplasty. All the studies showed a reduced risk of breast cancer with a relative risk varying from 0.2 to 0.7.

Boice and colleagues[25] showed a 28% reduction in breast cancer after reduction mammaplasty with greatest reduction in women 50 years and older. This study consisted of 31,901 women from the Swedish Inpatient Register undergoing reduction mammaplasty. The follow-up averaged 7.5 years and a 28% reduction in breast cancer risk was observed compared with a normal population. The greatest risk reduction was in women older than 50 and those followed for longer than 5 years.

SCREENING FOR BREAST CANCER AFTER REDUCTION MAMMAPLASTY

Muir and colleagues[26] reviewed more than 240,000 women undergoing screening mammography, 4743 had a previous reduction mammaplasty. Fewer cancers were detected in the breast reduction group with a relative risk of 0.71. There was no difference in recall rates for additional imaging between the 2 groups or significant differences in the pathologic type or location of cancers.

REFERENCES

1. American Society of Plastic Surgeons. 2014 Reconstructive plastic surgery statistics. 2014. Available at: http://www.plasticsurgery.org/Documents/news-resources/statistics/2014-statistics/reconstructive-procedure-trends-2014.pdf. Accessed June 24, 2015.
2. American Society of Plastic Surgeons. 2014 Cosmetic plastic surgery statistics. 2014. Available at: http://www.plasticsurgery.org/Documents/news-resources/statistics/2014-statistics/cosmetic-procedure-trends-2014.pdf. Accessed October 28, 2015.
3. Ambaye AB, MacLennan SE, Goodwin AJ, et al. Carcinoma and atypical hyperplasia in reduction mammaplasty: increased sampling leads to increased detection. A prospective study. Plast Reconstr Surg 2009;124(5):1386–92.
4. Clark CJ, Whang S, Paige KT. Incidence of precancerous lesions in breast reduction tissue: a pathologic review of 562 consecutive patients. Plast Reconstr Surg 2009;124(4):1033–9.
5. Cook IS, Fuller CE. Does histopathological examination of breast reduction specimens affect patient management and clinical follow up? J Clin Pathol 2004;57(3):286–9.
6. Ishag MT, Bashinsky DY, Beliaeva IV, et al. Pathologic findings in reduction mammaplasty specimens. Am J Clin Pathol 2003;120(3):377–80.
7. Tang CL, Brown MH, Levine R, et al. Breast cancer found at the time of breast reduction. Plast Reconstr Surg 1999;103(6):1682–6.
8. Colwell AS, Kukreja J, Breuing KH, et al. Occult breast carcinoma in reduction mammaplasty specimens: 14-year experience. Plast Reconstr Surg 2004;113(7):1984–8.
9. Hassan FE, Pacifico MD. Should we be analysing breast reduction specimens? A systematic analysis of over 1,000 consecutive cases. Aesthetic Plast Surg 2012;36(5):1105–13.
10. Sorin T, Fyad JP, Delay E, et al. Occult cancer in specimens of reduction mammaplasty aimed at symmetrization. A multicentric study of 2718 patients. Breast 2015;24(3):272–7.
11. Tadler M, Vlastos G, Pelte MF, et al. Breast lesions in reduction mammaplasty specimens: a histopathological pattern in 534 patients. Br J Cancer 2014;110(3):788–91.
12. Pharoah PD, Day NE, Duffy S, et al. Family history and the risk of breast cancer: a systematic review and meta-analysis. Int J Cancer 1997;71(5):800–9.
13. Chen S, Parmigiani G. Meta-analysis of BRCA1 and BRCA2 penetrance. J Clin Oncol 2007;25(11):1329–33.
14. Goodwin JT, Decroff C, Dauway E, et al. The management of incidental findings of reduction mammoplasty specimens. Can J Plast Surg 2013;21(4):226–8.
15. Page DL, Dupont WD, Rogers LW, et al. Atypical hyperplastic lesions of the female breast. A long-term follow-up study. Cancer 1985;55(11):2698–708.
16. Hennedige AA, Kong TY, Gandhi A. Oncological screening for bilateral breast reduction: a survey of practice variations in UK breast and plastics surgeons 2009. J Plast Reconstr Aesthet Surg 2011;64(7):878–83.
17. Ayhan S, Başterzi Y, Yavuzer R, et al. Histologic profiles of breast reduction specimens. Aesthetic Plast Surg 2002;26(3):203–5.
18. Pitanguy I, Torres E, Salgado F, et al. Breast pathology and reduction mammaplasty. Plast Reconstr Surg 2005;115(3):729–34 [discussion: 735].
19. The Royal College of Pathologists. Histopathology and cytoplathology of limited or no clinical value. 2nd edition. London: Royal College of Pathologists; 2005.
20. Desouki MM, Li Z, Hameed O, et al. Incidental atypical proliferative lesions in reduction mammoplasty specimens: analysis of 2498 cases from 2 tertiary women's health centers. Hum Pathol 2013;44(9):1877–81.
21. Dotto J, Kluk M, Geramizadeh B, et al. Frequency of clinically occult intraepithelial and invasive neoplasia in reduction mammoplasty specimens: a study of 516 cases. Int J Surg Pathol 2008;16(1):25–30.
22. Slezak S, Bluebond-Langner R. Occult carcinoma in 866 reduction mammaplasties: preserving the choice of lumpectomy. Plast Reconstr Surg 2011;127(2):525–30.
23. Spear SL, Rottman SJ, Seiboth LA, et al. Breast reconstruction using a staged nipple-sparing mastectomy following mastopexy or reduction. Plast Reconstr Surg 2012;129(3):572–81.
24. Tarone RE, Lipworth L, Young VL, et al. Breast reduction surgery and breast cancer risk: does

reduction mammaplasty have a role in primary prevention strategies for women at high risk of breast cancer? Plast Reconstr Surg 2004;113(7):2104–10 [discussion: 2111–2].

25. Boice JD Jr, Persson I, Brinton LA, et al. Breast cancer following breast reduction surgery in Sweden. Plast Reconstr Surg 2000;106(4):755–62.

26. Muir TM, Tresham J, Fritschi L, et al. Screening for breast cancer post reduction mammoplasty. Clin Radiol 2010;65(3):198–205.

27. Jansen DA, Murphy M, Kind GM, et al. Breast cancer in reduction mammoplasty: case reports and a survey of plastic surgeons. Plast Reconstr Surg 1998;101(2):361–4.

Avoiding the Unfavorable Outcome with Wise Pattern Breast Reduction

Juliana E. Hansen, MD

KEYWORDS

- Breast reduction • Reduction mammaplasty • Wise pattern • Inferior pedicle • Outcomes

KEY POINTS

- Design a Wise pattern with longer vertical limbs: 8 to 12 cm from nipple to inframammary fold.
- Limit undermining of skin flaps.
- Elevate skin flaps deep to the breast capsule to ensure perfusion.
- Create wide-based inferior pedicles.
- Establish tension-free closures by creating generous skin envelopes and performing a superficial fascial vertical closure.

INTRODUCTION

Wise pattern breast reduction remains the most popular method of performing moderate- to large-sized breast reductions in the United States. According to the American Board of Plastic Surgeons Maintenance of Certification tracer statistics from 2012, 83% of surgeons use a Wise pattern skin resection pattern for their primary technique. Despite the generalized acceptance that short scar techniques are good options for many patients and despite the universal desire to minimize scarring, the Wise pattern approach endures and remains widely taught and frequently used. This popularity is most likely because of the comfort level that surgeons have in applying this technique to all varieties and sizes of breast reductions and in achieving predictable results.

Inferior pedicle Wise pattern breast reductions have been criticized for creating flat boxy breasts that are prone to hypertrophic scarring from the ample scar burden. Without doubt, this technique may lead to these types of outcomes (**Fig. 1**). Often the most challenging patients are addressed using this standard technique though, and outcomes may be associated as much with the degree of difficulty of the case as with the technique used. Every case should be done, however, with the goal of obtaining an aesthetically pleasing result and this should be achievable. The Wise pattern inferior pedicle breast reduction it is not a bad operation; but it can, like any other method of reduction, be done badly.

Although this technique has endured, it has certainly evolved since the time that Dr Robert Wise first conceived of the brassiere pattern to facilitate breast reduction. As we consider ways to improve shape and outcomes and to minimize shape distortion, we should continually look for ways to modify the technique. Much can be learned from vertical techniques that can be applied to more traditional skin resection patterns and inferior pedicle techniques in order to improve outcomes.

The author has no financial or other conflicts of interest related to this topic or article.
Plastic and Reconstructive Surgery, Department of Surgery, Oregon Health and Science University, 3181 Southwest Sam Jackson Park Road, L352A, Portland, OR 97239, USA
E-mail address: hansenju@ohsu.edu

plasticsurgery.theclinics.com

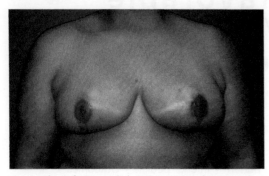

Fig. 1. The inferior pedicle Wise pattern breast reduction can result in a boxy shape to the lower pole of the breasts.

Although a Wise pattern skin resection always results in the traditional periareolar scar with a vertical limb along the breast meridian and an inframammary fold (IMF) scar, there is much variability in how that pattern is applied. Variables include nipple-areolar complex (NAC) height and diameter, vertical limb length, horizontal limb length, and the angle of divergence of the vertical limbs. Also, choice of pedicle may vary. Although the inferior pedicle is most commonly used, superomedial pedicles and free nipple graft techniques are also commonly used with the inverted T scar pattern.

Shape distortion after breast reduction can be a result of design flaw, execution of technique, or the result of postoperative complications. This article focuses primarily on optimal design and intraoperative techniques for prevention of shape distortion. By carefully considering the design of the skin resection pattern, choosing and designing an appropriate pedicle, preventing skin necrosis, and managing scars, shape distortion after Wise pattern breast reduction can be minimized.

HISTORICAL CONSIDERATIONS

The original Wise pattern, as described in 1956 by Robert Wise, MD used a plastic ring around the base of the breast to which a form, designed from various sized bra cups, was attached. The form was obtained from the makers of the Cordelia of Hollywood brassiere and was in fact a bra cup with the tip of the cone removed at the nipple position, opened along the 6:00 vertical of the standing cone. This form determined the skin pattern to be incised with the skin inferior to the pattern representing the skin to be excised. The parenchymal resection was aided by a second plastic form pattern, which secured the breast parenchyma

for an inferior wedge excision, resulting in a superior pedicle. There was no mention of de-epithelializing the skin around the NAC in the original description. The skin flaps were designed and modified by Wise specifically to reduce the rate of necrosis. His proposed technique created skin flaps with a more favorable length to width ratio and less undermining.[1–3]

Current Wise pattern breast reductions look very different than the original description. They are most commonly performed using an inferior pedicle. Superior pedicles and superomedial pedicles are also common though, particularly when a vertical breast reduction is converted intraoperatively into a Wise pattern to remove excess dog-ear skin at the base. Pedicle design is variable with regard to base width and the amount of parenchyma included with the pedicle. Skin de-epithelialization over the chosen pedicle is still common practice. This maneuver, designed to preserve the subdermal venous plexus and optimize perfusion, continues to be routine for most surgeons, though the need for this practice is not validated.[4]

The skin flap design varies widely depending on the length of the vertical limbs, angle of divergence of the vertical limbs, degree of undermining, and the length of the IMF incision. Use of the McKissock keyhole marker is a commonly used aid, whereas other surgeons, trained to freehand the marks, will always use a cut-as-you-go method. This method saves the NAC placement for the final stage of the procedure allowing for intraoperative modifications of the skin flaps as needed. Parenchymal management techniques may also vary widely, with some surgeons favoring internal shaping sutures and/or liposuction. The overall placement of the Wise pattern on the breast is variable, and nipple position and placement is subject to the surgeons' judgment. Considering this degree of variability, it is understandable that results can vary so greatly.

Aiming for consistent aesthetic results requires an understanding of the target. Ideal breast characteristics include a smooth, rounded lower pole of the breast, medial and lateral definition of the breast on the chest wall, a gradual slope and transition from the chest wall to the nipple, and an upper pole to lower pole ratio of 45:55.[5,6] Although not all patients' baseline characteristics lend themselves to creating the ideal aesthetic breast, every breast reduction should aim to achieve optimal aesthetic results. This outcome can be achieved in most cases by modifying the standards for traditional Wise pattern measurements as well as by tailoring all measurements to best match each patient's individual breast size, shape, and body habitus (**Fig. 2**).

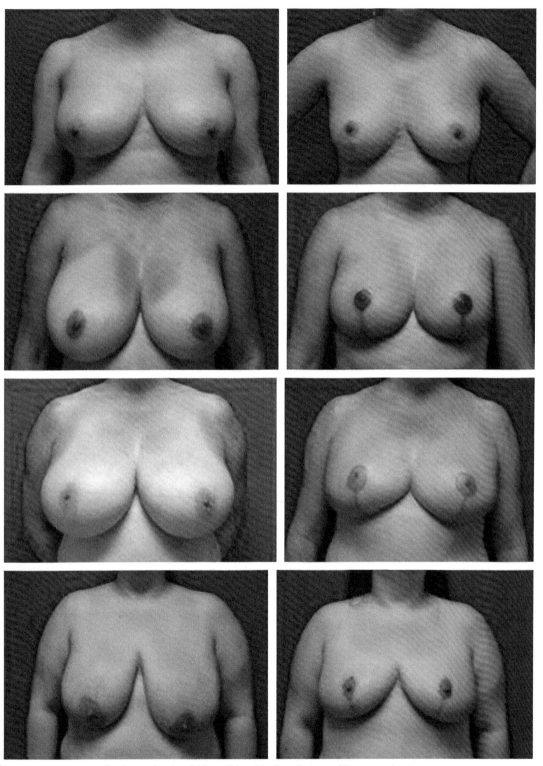

Fig. 2. Consistent aesthetic results should be achievable for all sizes of breast reductions.

DESIGNING SKIN FLAPS TO MINIMIZE SHAPE DISTORTION

Vertical limbs traditionally have been taught to be short, routinely with 5-cm limbs from the areola to the IMF. Short limbs of 4 to 5 cm were routinely used by some surgeons with the thought that less skin left behind prevents bottoming out and can prevent the nipple from being too high.[7,8] This thinking relies on the notion that the skin envelope is largely responsible for creating and maintaining the long-term shape of the breast. In contrast, the vertical breast reduction is based on the principle that the parenchymal pedicle design and position are responsible for creating shape and the skin envelope contours around the pedicle. It is this concept that supports much less skin resection overall in the vertical technique and no vertical skin resection at all. By incorporating these concepts into the Wise pattern design, new standards for limb lengths should be set. Vertical limbs should be designed routinely between 8 and 11 cm depending on the size of the patient (**Fig. 3**).

Short vertical limbs create a smaller skin envelope. In addition to resulting in a squared lower pole, the over-resection of skin leads to the need for more flap undermining and parenchymal resection. Traditionally, the upper skin flap was created by undermining up to the clavicle to allow for closure. This method creates skin flaps with a longer length to width ratio, which, when closed under tension, are more likely to undergo necrosis.

Additionally, when the skin envelope is too tight, the ability to close the breast after reduction depends on the amount of breast parenchyma that is removed. This situation can lead to over-resection of the parenchyma, resulting in suboptimal outcomes with breasts that lack projection and are disproportionately small.

Vertical limb length should be designed longer, with less skin resection, allowing for a more generous skin envelope, less need for undermining of the skin flaps, less tension on the closure, and the freedom to contour and sculpt the pedicle and the remaining breast parenchyma into the optimal shape.

Skin flap elevation should be done in a plane deep to the breast capsule and not subcutaneously. This plane will ensure skin flaps that have

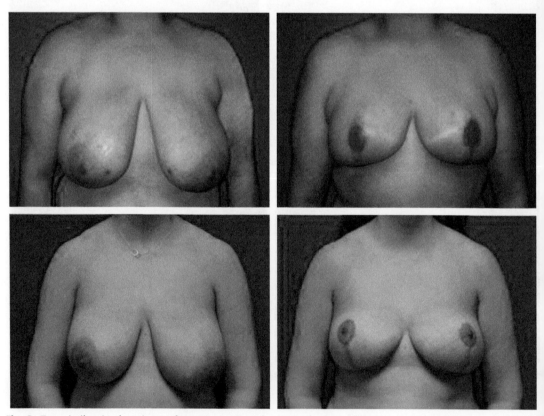

Fig. 3. Two similar-sized patients after Wise pattern breast reduction. The upper patient has vertical limbs of 5 cm. Longer, 10-cm vertical limb design in the lower patient can help to ensure a more rounded aesthetic result.

an axial pedicle rather than large random pattern flaps. The ideal plane for the superolateral flap should be deep to the course of the external mammary branch of the lateral thoracic artery. The lateral thoracic artery originates from the axillary artery and follows the lower border of the pectoralis minor muscle along the chest wall, supplying the pectoralis muscles and the serratus muscles. The external mammary branch, which comes off of the lateral thoracic artery, courses around the free edge of the pectoralis major muscle below the axilla to enter the breast, traveling deep to the breast capsule.

In the superomedial skin flap, the plane should be deep to the course of the second intercostal artery.

The internal thoracic artery (internal mammary) has multiple perforating branches in addition to the segmental intercostal branches. The second through fourth intercostal spaces have the largest perforating branches, which hypertrophy to accommodate the growing breast, particularly during pregnancy and lactation. These perforating branches leave the chest wall 2 to 3 cm lateral to the edge of the sternum, running deep to the breast capsule to supply the breast and the skin. These branches course toward the NACs, entering on the right side at approximately 1:00 and on the left side at approximately 11:00.

Although most surgeons try to elevate thick skin flaps, the patients' body habitus, degree of distinct breast capsule, volume of planned parenchymal resection, and degree of fat relative to breast stroma can make the plane for skin flap elevation quite variable. Traditionally, skin flaps were taught to be at least 1 cm thick, focusing on overall thickness rather than the optimal plane. Natural variation in patients' body habitus and breast quality requires a focus on depth into the correct plane rather than a standard thickness.

In older patients or patients with primarily fatty breasts, the breast capsule may not be as distinct. Establishing an overly thick plane at the outset of the elevation will help to ensure that these vessels are captured. As the skin flaps are elevated, it is not uncommon for the flap thickness to vary. Inadvertent transition into the subcutaneous plane proximally, which damages either of these vessels, may increase the incidence of skin flap necrosis.

The upper outer quadrant of the breast has the most breast tissue present. In the particularly dense breast, it is common and usual to remove all of the platelike breast tissue that is present in that location. Aggressive excision, however, may damage the descending external mammary branch as it enters the breast at the lateral border of the pectoralis minor muscle.[9] In all patients, an awareness of the anatomic course and thoughtful preservation of the pedicles for the skin flaps will ensure that they are robust, minimizing complications.

Undermining should be limited to the upper point of ligamentous breast attachments to the skin. Minimal undermining will result in better perfusion; but if the upper pole ligaments are not released, it can affect the contour of the upper pole. The aesthetic breast should maintain a straight upper pole with a gradual slope from the clavicle to the nipple. The nipples should project from the anterior-most point of the breast with a neutral or slight upward angulation. If there are tight upper pole ligaments, which are not released, the slope from the clavicle to the nipple becomes an acute angle with an abrupt takeoff from the chest wall (**Fig. 4**).

CREATING THE PEDICLE TO MINIMIZE SHAPE DISTORTION

The traditional inferior pedicle was tongue shaped and considered to be more of a dermal pedicle.[10] The pedicle instead should be designed with the long-term shape in mind. The ideal aesthetic breast demonstrates a straight upper pole without an angled takeoff of the breast from the chest wall. In seeking to create these ideal characteristics, limited resection of parenchyma from the upper chest can help to prevent concavity. The optimal shape after any technique of breast reduction will be obtained by focusing more on what is left behind than what is removed.

The inferior pedicle should be designed with a wide horizontal and vertical base of 8 to 10 cm. The pedicle should be created by strongly beveling the skin and breast tissue to be resected away from the base of the pedicle, which will prevent scalloping. As the sculpting of the pedicle moves toward the nipple, there is tapering of the bevel to result in a pyramid of parenchyma with the NAC at the apex and pointing forward (**Fig. 5**).

CLOSURE

Thicker skin flaps with breast parenchyma included are heartier and allow for closure of the breast capsule. This superficial fascial closure is an important factor in providing internal support and preventing lower pole stretch or bottoming out. Anatomic fascial closure is only feasible along the vertical limbs when performing an inferior pedicle breast reduction but is sufficient in providing structural support and reducing tension on the skin closure (**Fig. 6**). A tension-free vertical closure will result in improved scarring along the

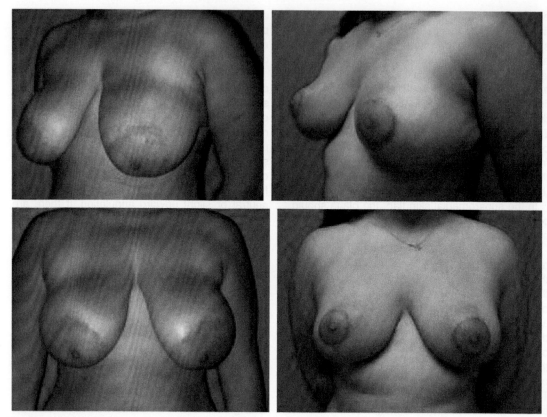

Fig. 4. Inadequate release of tight upper pole ligaments will result in upper pole angle deformities.

vertical closure. This combination of a wide-based pyramidal inferior pedicle, which preserves much of the upper pole parenchyma with a horizontal fascial sling for internal support, will create optimal and long-lasting breast shape while preventing significant lower pole descent (**Fig. 7**).

A combination of deeper support sutures and subcuticular sutures should be used for all sites of closure. The inset of the NAC can be particularly prone to visible suture marks and permanent unacceptable scarring from external sutures (**Fig. 8**).

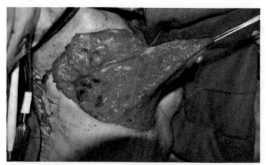

Fig. 5. Inferior pedicles designed with a wide-based pyramidal shape will maintain upper pole fullness and allow for improved shape.

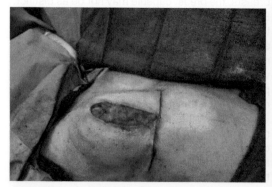

Fig. 6. Closure of the superficial fascia along the vertical closure can help provide internal support and take tension off the skin closure.

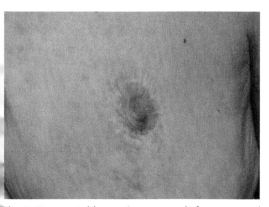

Fig. 7. Unacceptable scarring can result from external sutures on the nipple-areolar inset.

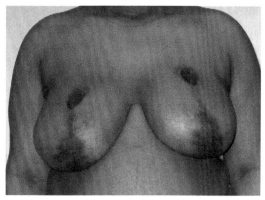

Fig. 9. Careful attention to nipple placement and prevention of excessive bottoming out can prevent nipple malposition.

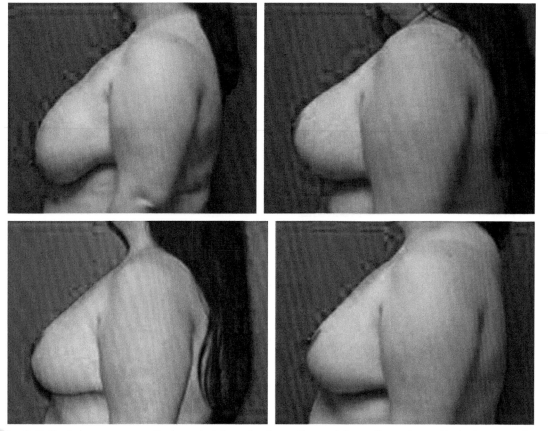

Fig. 8. Patient shown preoperatively and at 6 weeks, 3 months, and 4 months postoperatively demonstrating maintenance of upper pole shape and minimal bottoming out.

NIPPLE POSITION

Shape distortion can be prevented and aesthetic results optimized by focusing on the ideal placement of the NAC. The ultimate appearance will be affected not only by the absolute height and position of the NAC relative to the sternal notch but also by the relative position of the nipple on the breast after skin relaxation and parenchymal settling (**Fig. 9**). Without doubt the nipple that is too high will create the most distressing result for patients, creating areolar show in a bra or a bathing suit. The nipple that is positioned too low will not, at least, create new problems but may not create optimal aesthetic results.

Ideal nipple position should be patient specific, determined after assessing all available standards and measurements. These measurements include a sternal notch to nipple distance of 20 to 23 cm, just above midhumeral height, 2 cm above the

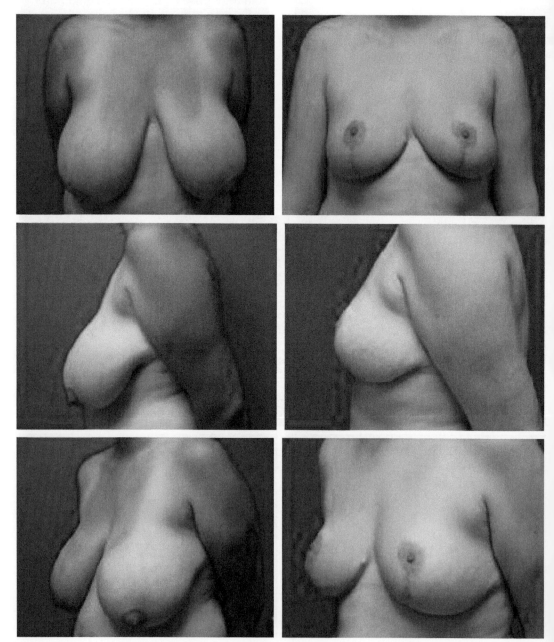

Fig. 10. Careful initial placement of nipples and internal support of the lower pole will maintain ideal nipple position and breast proportions even after large reductions.

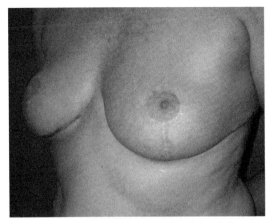

Fig. 11. This patient demonstrated well-healed periareolar and vertical scars with hypertrophic IMF scars.

IMF, 10 cm below the upper chest wall border of the breast, or 5 to 7 cm below the axillary fold. Using the techniques of a wide-based pyramidal inferior pedicle, generous skin flaps closed without tension, and superficial fascial closure, the nipple can be set with confidence at an aesthetic height without concern that the breast will bottom out with time, resulting in an imbalance in the nipple-areolar position relative to the breast (**Fig. 10**).

MANAGING SCARS TO OPTIMIZE OUTCOMES

Scar management should be a routine component of any breast reduction, particularly when there are inframammary scars, which seem to be prone to hypertrophy (**Fig. 11**). Postoperative scar management should begin by 2 weeks after surgery, during the proliferative phase of wound healing, and continue into the remodeling phase for at least 2 months. Silicone gel sheeting has been found to be an effective measure for preventing scar hypertrophy.[11–13]

POSTOPERATIVE REVISION

Management of the unfavorable result after Wise pattern breast reduction generally focuses on the IMF. Medial and lateral resection along the fold can improve a squared contour, greatly improving the postoperative aesthetic results. Nipple position that is too high is also most safely and effectively treated by lower pole wedge resection. Although this will not lengthen the sternal notch to nipple distance, this will provide improved balance to the breast and improved proportions (**Fig. 12**).

SUMMARY POINTS FOR AVOIDING THE UNFAVORABLE OUTCOME WITH WISE PATTERN BREAST REDUCTION

It is the execution of the well-planned design that will ultimately determine the outcome of the procedure. Pedicle and skin flap design should be created with a focus more on what is left behind than what is removed. Skin flaps can be elevated as pedicled, robust flaps and the inferior pedicle as a wide-based, sculpted pyramid. With this mind-set, one can control breast shape and healing better and optimize outcomes.

- Wise pattern design with longer vertical limbs: 8 to 12 cm from nipple to IMF
- Limited undermining of skin flaps
- Elevation of skin flaps deep to the breast capsule
- Tension-free closures, facilitated by generous skin envelopes, superficial fascial vertical closures, and thick skin flaps
- Routine scar management with silicone gel sheeting

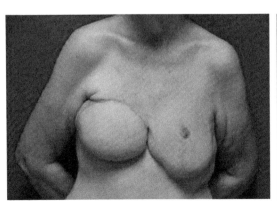
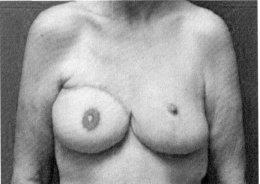

Fig. 12. Lower pole resection of the left breast after prior reduction improves the relative nipple position.

REFERENCES

1. Wise RJ. A preliminary report on a method of planning the mammaplasty. Plast Reconstr Surg 1956; 17:367–75.

2. Wise RJ, Gannon JP, Hill JR. Further experience with reduction mammaplasty. Plast Reconstr Surg 1963; 32:12–20.

3. Wise J. Treatment of breast hypertrophy. Clin Plast Surg 1976;3(2):289–300.

4. Iwuagwu OC, Drew PJ. Deskinning versus deepithelialization for inferior pedicle reduction mammoplasty: a prospective comparative analysis. Aesthetic Plast Surg 2005;29:202–4.

5. Mallucci P, Branford OA. Population analysis of the perfect breast: a morphometric analysis. Plast Reconstr Surg 2014;134:436–47.

6. Mallucci P, Branford OA. Concepts in aesthetic breast dimensions: analysis of the ideal breast. J Plast Reconstr Aesthet Surg 2012;65:8–16.

7. Courtiss EH, Goldwyn RM. Reduction mammaplasty by the inferior pedicle technique. Plast Reconstr Surg 1977;59:500–7.

8. Hidalgo DA. Improving safety and aesthetic results in inverted T scar breast reduction. Plast Reconstr Surg 1999;103:874–86.

9. Gray H. The axillary artery. In: Goss CM, editor. Anatomy of the human body. Philadelphia: Lea and Febiger; 1959. p. 654–5.

10. McKissock PK. Reduction mammaplasty with a vertical dermal flap. Plast Reconstr Surg 1971;49:245–52.

11. Cruz-Korchin NI. Effectiveness of silicone sheets in the prevention of hypertrophic breast scars. Ann Plast Surg 1996;37:345–8.

12. Fulton JE Jr. Silicone gel sheeting for the prevention and management of evolving hypertrophic and keloid scars. Dermatol Surg 1995;21:947–51.

13. Gauglitz GG, Korting HC, Pavicic T, et al. Hypertrophic scarring and keloids: pathomechanisms and current and emerging treatment strategies. Mol Med 2011;17(1–2):113–25.

Managing Complications in Vertical Mammaplasty

Marta Misani, MD[a],*, Albert De Mey, MD[b]

KEYWORDS

- Vertical scar mammaplasty • Superior pedicle breast reduction • Lejour technique
- Breast reduction complications

KEY POINTS

- A precise examination of patient is necessary for the choice of the surgical technique.
- Medical history and patient habits are important prognostic factors of any complications.
- Mastering a surgical technique and examining the results of its application is the starting point to improve the technique and reduce complications.

INTRODUCTION

In 1989, Professor Lejour introduced a new technique of vertical scar breast reduction,[1] which immediately gained popularity and nowadays represents a standard technique worldwide. The most innovative aspect of her technique was the vertical-only scar, which had a double purpose: a more aesthetic outcome, thanks to the reduced scar length, and fewer scar-related complications.[2–4]

In our center, where Professor Lejour is the former chief of the Plastic and Reconstructive Surgery Department, we immediately adopted the technique and over the years we have modified it by reducing vertical pillars skin undermining, avoiding systematic liposuction, using a superomedial pedicle in large breasts, and adding a horizontal skin resection at the end of the procedure if necessary.[5]

Recently, we analyzed all breast reduction procedures performed between 1991 and 2013 in our center, and we were able to evaluate complications and their management, and we have improved our technique to make it reproducible for all trainees. We share herein our experience and focus on the management of complications of the vertical scar mammaplasty.

PATIENTS AND TECHNIQUE SELECTION

Breast reduction has become a very common surgical procedure. It represents nowadays the most performed operation in our institution among general plastic surgery procedures. A good clinical history and physical examination are the key points to a successful breast reduction. Anamnesis has its critical points: history of smoking, diabetes, and a high body mass index (BMI) being the main negative factors affecting wound healing. Age is an important factor in choosing the surgical technique, as well as previous pregnancies. In the vast majority of cases, we use a superior areolar pedicle and vertical scar technique. When faced with a larger breast with high BMI and severe ptosis, we are moving to a superomedial areolar pedicle and a short submammary scar or nipple–areola complex graft.

THE MODIFIED LEJOUR TECHNIQUE

The Lejour technique is based on a superior pedicle, on which the blood supply of the areola relies and a central glandular resection, with central suturing of the medial and lateral pillars. The skin is undermined on the vertical scar and the excess skin at the bottom of the scar is sutured

[a] CHR Mons Hainaut, 7000 Mons, Belgium; [b] Clinique du Parc Léopold, Rue Froissart 38, 1040 Brussels, Belgium
* Corresponding author.
E-mail address: martamisani@gmail.com

Clin Plastic Surg 43 (2016) 359–363
http://dx.doi.org/10.1016/j.cps.2015.12.014
0094-1298/16/$ – see front matter © 2016 Elsevier Inc. All rights reserved.

plasticsurgery.theclinics.com

by rippling the skin to reduce vertical length.[1] In addition, liposuction has been integrated into the procedure, to better shape the breast, performed for the first time in this kind of surgery.[2]

Since its original description, the technique of superior pedicle vertical scar mammaplasty has been modified, allowing plastic surgeons to benefit from the advantages of this technique while avoiding some associated unfavorable results.[4] The modifications that were brought to the technique were essentially a reduction of the skin undermining, limiting or avoiding liposuction, avoiding tight glandular stitches, and adding a small horizontal scar for very large breasts at the end of the operation.[6,7]

TECHNIQUE, MATERIALS, AND METHODS

We recently carried on a review on the evolution of the technique, complications and outcomes comparing 3 periods: 1991 to 1996, 1996 to 2007[8] and 2008 to 2013. This cohort includes a series of 1030 consecutive patients who underwent operations at the University Hospital Brugmann, Brussels. The study consisted of a review of the medical charts. The modified Lejour technique with only a vertical scar was used in 57% of our patients and a short horizontal scar was added in 43% of the patients operated between 2008 and 2013.

Patient characteristics (age and BMI) and factors possibly associated with an increased risk of postoperative complications such as diabetes and smoking, were recorded. The weight of the resection for each breast (in grams), the elevation of the nipple–areola complex, and the experience of the surgeon (senior: graduated plastic surgeon, junior: surgeon in training) were recorded.

During the operation, all patients were given a dose of antibiotics (amoxicillin and clavulanic acid or cephazolin), which was continued for 24 hours postoperatively. A suction drain was inserted through the scar or through a separated incision in the anterior axillary line. The wound dressing was changed 48 hours after the surgery and the drains were removed when it collected less than 30 mL/d. After leaving the hospital, all patients were seen in consultation every week during the first month and then after 3, 6, 12, 24, and 36 months. The stitches were removed at 3 weeks postoperatively.

COMPLICATIONS

Postoperative complications were divided into 2 groups: minor and major. Superficial wound dehiscence, inferior skin and fat excess, hematoma, seroma partial areolar necrosis, inverted, nipple and loss of sensation were considered minor complications. Glandular infection, total areolar necrosis, and glandular necrosis were considered major complications. During the study period, the overall rate of complications decreased from 45% to 26%. The need for secondary correction decreased from 22% to 16%. The main risk factors for major complications were greater BMI and the amount of glandular resection. For minor complications, smoking and the experience of the surgeon were significant.[5]

Minor Complications

The main complications observed in our series were superficial would dehiscence (**Fig. 1**) and skin and fat excess. Superficial would dehiscence is a common complication in all breast reduction techniques.[8] It is strongly associated with skin undermining of excessive tension, but also with patient characteristics, especially of factor affecting wound healing as well as a high BMI. It is well-known that a history of tobacco smoking can affect wound healing; this is owing to alterations in the microcirculation of the sutured skin edges. To avoid this problem, we currently ask people to stop smoking, or at least reduce tobacco consumption, at least 3 weeks before surgery. Diabetes is another important factor compromising skin healing and increasing the risk of infection. For these patients, a prolonged administration of antibiotic prophylaxis sometimes is recommended.

From a technical point of view, we now limit the skin undermining along the vertical scar and avoid a massive puckering of the skin by a tight suture. Hematomas and seromas are nonspecific complications of the vertical scar mammaplasty. However, in the original technique, a large liposuction of the breast led to 30% of postoperative seromas and 12% of hematomas. A more gentle handling of the breast tissue and limiting the liposuction to small areas of the lower pole at the end of the operation reduced the incidence of seroma to 2% and hematomas to 3%.

In some large resections of soft fatty breasts, an inverted nipple has been observed in rare cases. This complication was always owing to an excessive anchoring of the areolar pedicle to the pectoral muscle at the upper pole of the breast. This outcome could be avoided by a careful suture of the glandular pillars only starting at the deep upper pole of the gland.

Excess skin and fat is an unfavorable result strongly related to the surgical technique.[9] In our series, we noticed that the incidence of this complication was substantially reduced with the insertion

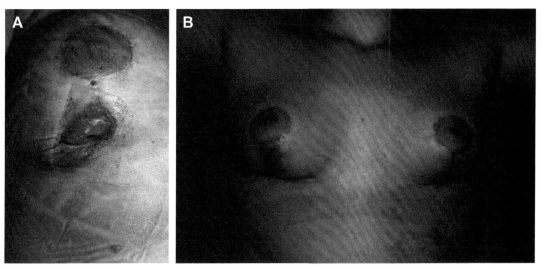

Fig. 1. (A) Superficial wound dehiscence of the vertical scar. (B) Conservative treatment of wound dehiscence.

of a small horizontal scar in the submammary fold at the end of the operation (**Fig. 2**). This resection is always decided only at the end of the operation when the surgeon realize that the elasticity of the skin will not be sufficient to absorb the skin excess with a purse string suture. When designed at the end of the operation, the horizontal submammary scar is always well-positioned and shorter that it would have been if drawn before the operation. This procedure was required in 43% of our series of 325 patients. However, we still had to perform

6% secondary submammary fold corrections, always under local anesthesia. Postoperative remaining fat excess is less common, because it can be easily managed by liposuction in the lower quadrants of the breast after modeling the gland.

Partial areolar necrosis is another minor complication we have to deal with. It is strongly related to the thickness and width of the pedicle, together with a history of tobacco smoking. It is seldom owing to a reduction of the arterial supply, but in most of the cases by a venous congestion. In large

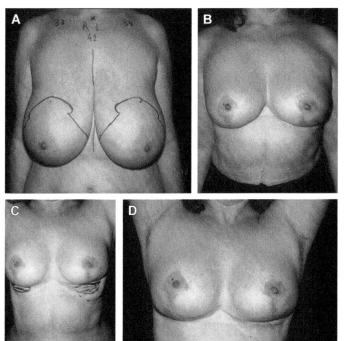

Fig. 2. (A) Drawing of a classical vertical scar mammaplasty. (B) Immediate postoperative results of vertical scar mammaplasty. (C) At 6 months postoperatively, there remains excess skin at the inferior part of the vertical scar. (D) Correction of excess skin by adding a short horizontal scar.

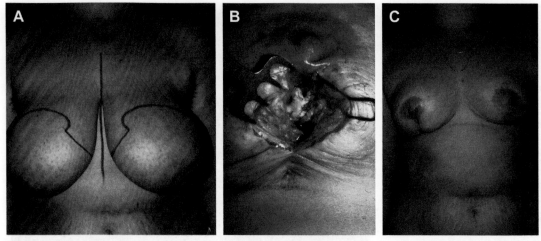

Fig. 3. (*A*) Preoperative drawings. (*B*) Vertical scar dehiscence with liponecrosis treated surgically by debridement. (*C*) The results at 6 months after surgical debridement of vertical dehiscence.

breasts, however, we use a superomedial pedicle with a wider basis.[10] In case of an impaired venous return, we recommend to release all the periareolar sutures. Fortunately, in most cases, the result is only a temporary superficial epidermolysis, which presents with blisters and resolved rapidly with local dressings. If the defect represents more than one-half the areola surface, we do not hesitate to debride it and reconstruct a new nipple–areola complex with a split thickness skin graft followed by a skin tattoo.

Finally, loss of nipple–areolar sensation has been reported often. In a prospective study, we demonstrated that none of our breasts was insensate.[11] However, in large resections, pressure recovery was obtained after 1 year but vibration and temperature sensation were absent in several cases after resection of more than 1 kg of tissue per breast.

Major Complications

Major complications include those that compromise the aesthetic results of the intervention, and that often require a second surgery or hospitalization. The incidence rate is lower than that of minor complications, but surgeons need to treat them when they arise. In our series, we improved their occurrence to less than 2% with the modifications discussed.

Complete areolar necrosis is the most common major complication. It is owing, like partial necrosis, to reduced blood supply to the areola. As described for partial areolar necrosis, this reduced supply may be owing to an inappropriate surgical technique or preoperative drawings. Complete areolar necrosis always requires surgical treatment, which consists of precise debridement and

reconstruction of the new nipple–areola complex by skin graft and a tattoo.

Glandular infection and glandular necrosis have a substantial impact on aesthetic results. This complication is not only owing to a too aggressive procedure, but in the majority of cases observed in patients with a high BMI or after resection of more than 1 kg of tissue. Treatment includes appropriate antibiotic coverage and prompt debridement of necrotic tissue. The debridement should be followed by a remodeling of the gland to achieve a pleasing aesthetic result (**Fig. 3**).

SUMMARY

By reviewing the charts of more than 1000 patients who underwent breast reduction with a vertical scar in the Brugmann University Hospital between 1991 and 2013, we have evaluated the effects of the modifications proposed along the years to the original Lejour technique. The improved results were obtained by a gentle handling of the breast tissue and adding a short submammary scar in nearly 50% of our cases at the end of the operation. The greatest risk factor for complication remains, as in any surgery, a BMI of more than 30 kg/m², resection of more than 1 kg of tissue per breast, and the patient's smoking habits.

REFERENCES

1. Lejour M. Vertical mammoplasty and liposuction of the breast. Plast Reconstr Surg 1994;94(1):100–14.
2. Lejour M. Vertical mammaplasty and liposuction. St Louis (MO): Quality Medical Publishing; 1994.
3. Lejour M. Vertical mammaplasty: early complications after 250 personal consecutive cases. Plast Reconstr Surg 1999;104(3):764–70.

4. Lejour M. Vertical mammaplasty: update and appraisal of late results. Plast Reconstr Surg 1999; 104:771–81.

5. Berthe JV, Massaut J, Greuse M, et al. The vertical mammaplasty: a reappraisal of the technique and its complications. Plast Reconstr Surg 2003;111(7): 2192–9 [discussion 2200 2].

6. Yukesel F, Karago H, Sever C, et al. Experience with vertical mammaplasty: advantages and drawbacks of Hall-Findlay's superomedial pedicle technique and improving the results by adding modifications to the technique. Aesthetic Plast Surg 2012;36: 1329–33.

7. Azzam C, De Mey A. Vertical scar mammaplasty in gigantomastia: retrospective study of 115 patients treated using the modified Lejour technique. Aesthetic Plast Surg 2007;31(3):294–8.

8. Zoumaras J, Lawrence J. Inverted T versus vertical scar breast reduction: one surgeon's 5 year experience with consecutive patients. Aesthet Surg J 2008;28:521–6.

9. Beer GM, Spicher I, Cierpka KA, et al. Benefits and pitfalls of vertical scar breast reduction. Br J Plast Surg 2004;57:12–9.

10. Rinker B. Lowering revision rates in medial pedicle breast reduction by the selective addition of " inverted T" technique. Aesthetic Plast Surg 2013;37:341.

11. Greuse M, Hamdi M, De Mey A. Breast sensitivity after vertical mammaplasty. Plast Reconstr Surg 2001;107:970–6.

The Short Scar Periareolar Inferior Pedicle Reduction Mammaplasty
Management of Complications

Dennis C. Hammond, MD*, Kuylhee Kim, MD

KEYWORDS

• SPAIR • Breast reduction • Complications

KEY POINTS

- The skin pattern of the short scar periareolar inferior pedicle reduction mammaplasty creates inequality in the incision lengths around the periareolar and vertical incisions.
- This inequality can lead to delayed wound healing, widened or unattractive scars, and shape distortion.
- Based on an inferior pedicle, blood supply issues to the nipple-areolar complex are rare.
- The overall complication rate is low, and the aesthetic results are excellent.

INTRODUCTION

Breast reduction is one of the most common plastic surgery procedures performed on the breast.[1] Over time, several different approaches to this operation have been described, each designed to variably provide the potential for more aesthetic breast shapes, reduced scars, and decreased complication rates. As a result, there are now numerous alternatives to the standard inverted-T inferior pedicle technique. The short scar periareolar inferior pedicle reduction (SPAIR) mammaplasty is one of these techniques.[2–7] Originally, the procedure was designed to reduce the scar burden associated with breast reduction. However, as experience with the technique grew, it became evident that the aesthetic results were of high quality and the degree of postoperative shape change over time was not as dramatic as can happen with the inverted-T procedure. However, as with any operative procedure, postoperative complications can occur. The purpose of this article is to outline these potential complications that are of particular concern with the SPAIR mammaplasty and describe methods for their treatment and prevention.

TECHNIQUE

By way of reference, the SPAIR mammaplasty is based on an inferior pedicle to provide vascularity to the nipple-areolar complex (NAC). The underlying breast septum is also preserved to enhance the viability of the pedicle.[8] The redundant tissue is resected from around the pedicle creating a U-shaped block of tissue. The skin pattern uses a circumvertical approach whereby the medial and lateral breast flaps are brought around and under the inferior pedicle to close off the vertical segment and help cone the breast. This maneuver

Disclosures: Dr D.C. Hammond receives royalties related to the sale of the book *Atlas of Aesthetic Breast Surgery* published by Elsevier, 2009.
Partners in Plastic Surgery, 4070 Lake Drive, Suite 202, Grand Rapids, MI 49546, USA
* Corresponding author.
E-mail address: drhammond@pipsmd.com

Clin Plastic Surg 43 (2016) 365–372
http://dx.doi.org/10.1016/j.cps.2015.12.010
0094-1298/16/$ – see front matter © 2016 Elsevier Inc. All rights reserved.

creates a vertical scar that runs down from the NAC and variably courses inferolaterally to the inframammary fold (IMF). Finally the NAC is inset into the pattern using an interlocking purse-string suture (**Fig. 1**).[9]

COMPLICATIONS
Standard Operative Complications

All of the usual complications associated with breast reduction are also potentially associated with the SPAIR mammaplasty, including infection, hematoma, seroma, delayed wound healing, loss of nipple sensation, ischemia or necrosis of the NAC, rehypertrophy, asymmetry, and shape distortion. However, because of a unique combination of tissue management strategies, there are several potential complications that can be of particular concern when using the SPAIR.

Delayed wound healing

Delayed wound healing is the most common complication associated with the SPAIR mammaplasty. Although any portion of the incision pattern can experience wound breakdown with postoperative dehiscence, this most commonly occurs

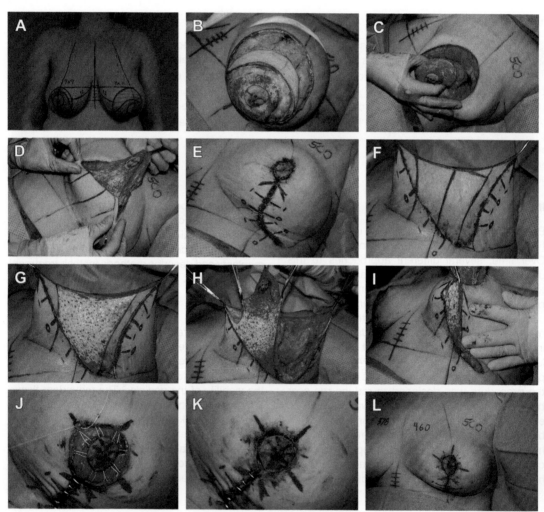

Fig. 1. (*A*) Preoperative marking in preparation for an SPAIR mammaplasty. (*B*) The areolar and periareolar incisions are made, and the inferior pedicle is de-epithelized. (*C*) A horseshoe-shaped segment of breast parenchyma is resected from around the inferior pedicle. (*D, E*) The vertical plication line can be set by progressively tailor tracking the skin edges together until a pleasing shape is created. (*F*) Appearance of vertical segment after removal of the staples. (*G, H*) The inferior pedicle is de-epithelized. The lateral flap is released from the pedicle. (*I*) The medial and lateral flaps are brought together to complete the vertical closure. (*J*) An interlocking Teflon suture is placed to control the periareolar defect. (*K*) Appearance of the areola after cinching down of the interlocking suture. (*L*) Final appearance.

along the midaspect of the vertical incision where the tension on the wound is the greatest. Typically patients present at approximately 1 week postoperatively with a variably sized opening with serous drainage. Treatment is conservative, as the wound will heal secondarily over a period of 2 to 4 weeks (**Fig. 2**). Only in cases of significant dehiscence is debridement and reclosure attempted (**Fig. 3**).

Fat necrosis

It is difficult to assess the viability of the fatty portion of the breast at the time of reduction, and devascularized tissues only become evident later on when the dead fat becomes encapsulated by scar. Such areas present as a rounded palpable mass usually present above the NAC, as this represents the terminal end of the pedicle that is farthest away from the blood supply. When this complication occurs, initial treatment consists of observation as resolution of edema and absorption of the necrotic fat can occur resulting in disappearance of the mass. If a mass persists up to a year postoperatively, biopsy and removal is recommended simply to avoid any potential for delay in diagnosis should an actual tumor ever develop.

Late seroma scar contracture

Often an unrecognized seroma can develop postoperatively that actually contributes to a full, rounded, and aesthetic shape during the early postoperative period. However, in selected cases, as the seroma resolves, the seroma cavity contracts creating a tethering force on the surrounding breast and NAC. Patients then present at approximately the 6-week mark with flattening of the breast, loss of projection, and a distorted shape with peripheral rounding and excess upper pole fullness. If the degree of contracture is mild, simple observation will allow settling of the tissues to occur and the shape and projection will improve over time. However, in more severe cases, the contracture can lead to a significant and long-lasting distortion in breast shape. Operative intervention at the 6- to 12-month mark is focused on redoing the scars and redeveloping the peripedicle dissection where the remnants of the seroma cavity can be identified coursing deeply around the superior aspect of the inferior pedicle. With simple excision of the scar and placement of a drain, the contracture is completely removed and the shape of the breast restored. During the revision of the scars, the old interlocking Teflon suture is removed and a new periareolar suture is applied to control the NAC. Any attempt to accomplish the dissection without removing the old periareolar suture limits the exposure too significantly and can result in distortion of the NAC postoperatively (**Fig. 4**).

Shape distortion

One of the hallmarks of the SPAIR mammaplasty is maintenance of shape postoperatively. As a result of the maintenance of the attachments along the IMF that occurs during the dissection of the flaps and the pedicle, the position of the IMF does not move. However, as with all breast reduction techniques, by dissecting a pedicle and removing the redundant tissue, the inherent fascial support structure (Cooper ligaments) of the breast is interrupted. This interruption predisposes to postoperative skin stretch with variable loss of breast shape. This loss tends to be noted more with

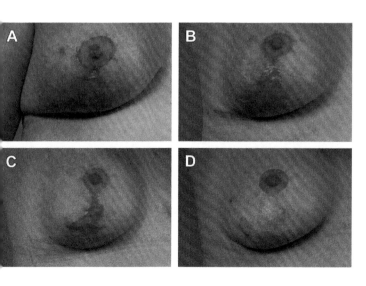

Fig. 2. (*A*) Wound breakdown at the midportion of the vertical segment 3 weeks after breast reduction using the SPAIR technique. The patient was treated by only conservative observation without any surgical intervention. (*B*) One month later, the wound is totally healed. (*C*) Six-month postoperative appearance. (*D*) The 18-month postoperative result showing stable wound healing with an acceptable appearance of the scar.

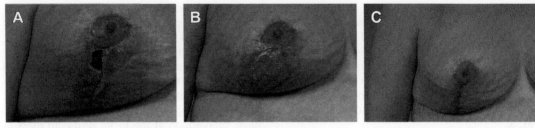

Fig. 3. (*A*) Delayed wound healing on the vertical segment 3 weeks after breast reduction using the SPAIR technique. A black necrotic eschar was noticed in the proximal portion, and dehiscence developed along half of the vertical incision (*B*). The necrotic tissue was debrided, and the defect was closed under local anesthesia resulting in stable wound healing at 4 weeks (*C*).

heavier breasts or in patients who have had massive weight loss. Fortunately, the operative correction is very straightforward and does not involve any new scars. By simply reapplying the circumvertical pattern, not only can the redundant skin envelope be taken up with improvement in breast shape but also the scars can be revised, often leading to a less noticeable appearance (**Fig. 5**).

Asymmetry

Asymmetry after SPAIR mammaplasty can occur with regard to the shape or size of the breast or with the position of the NAC. Fortunately, such asymmetries are easily treated with simple

reapplication of the circumvertical pattern. By differentially taking up the skin along the vertical, periareolar, or both incision patterns, almost any asymmetry can be improved in a simple fashion without the need to add any new scars. This fact makes revision a very rewarding undertaking as outstanding results can be reliably and predictably obtained.

Nipple-areolar complex distortion

Because of the forces placed on the areolar closure, distortion in the shape and size of the areola can occur postoperatively. Also, if the discrepancy between the dimensions of the areolar and periareolar incisions becomes too

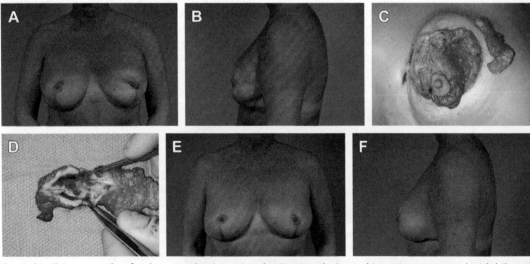

Fig. 4. (*A*, *B*) Four months after breast reduction using the SPAIR technique, this patient presented with bilateral contracted and distorted breasts. The breasts showed an excessive upper pole fullness along with irregular contours with the NAC being tethered down to the deeply situated seroma cavity and surrounding scar. (*C*) At surgery, a contracted seroma cavity was removed from around the top of the inferior pedicle along with the associated tethering scar. (*D*) When the scarred seroma cavity was opened, the residual seroma space could be visualized. (*E*, *F*) Six-month postoperative appearance shows a natural shape of breast without any contraction or surface irregularity.

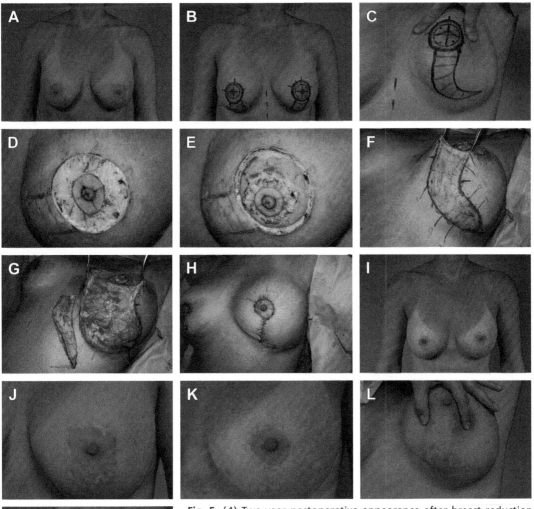

Fig. 5. (*A*) Two-year postoperative appearance after breast reduction. The NACs are distorted and asymmetric, and the skin of the lower pole is hypopigmented as a result of delayed wound healing. (*B, C*) Preoperative marking in preparation for revision using the circumvertical pattern. (*D*) After making the areolar and periareolar incisions, the intervening skin is de-epithelized. (*E*) The dermis around the periareolar opening is divided leaving a small dermal cuff. This cuff will eventually hold the Teflon suture. (*F*) The dimension of the vertical segment. (*G*) The redundant vertical skin and scar are removed as a full-thickness segment. (*H*) Final result. (*I*) Seven-month postoperative result showing the improvement in the shape of the breast. (*J, K*) The improvement in the appearance of the areola. (*L, M*) The vertical scar.

great, persistent pleating around the periareolar scar can fail to completely resolve. In these instances, a simple redo of the periareolar closure using the interlocking technique[4] can remove the pleating, reduce the size of the areola, and create a circular areolar shape with a fine-line scar. This technique can also be applied to other types of cases whereby any type of periareolar closure that resulted in a less than desired result

can be improved. With precise preoperative planning and then control of the periareolar opening using the interlocking technique, tremendous improvement in all types of cases can be realized (**Fig. 6**).

Areolar herniation

As a result of the forces applied by the interlocking suture around the areola, the underlying breast can

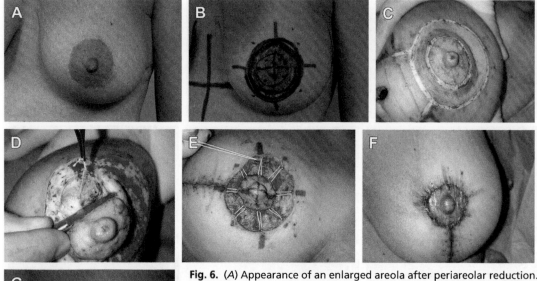

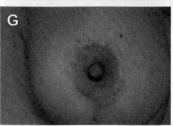

Fig. 6. (*A*) Appearance of an enlarged areola after periareolar reduction. (*B*) Marks in preparation for a revision using the interlocking technique. (*C*) The areolar and periareolar incisions are made. (*D*) The old Teflon suture is removed. (*E*) Appearance after placement of the interlocking suture. (*F*) Immediate postoperative appearance. (*G*) Appearance after 6 months shows a stable and reduced areolar diameter.

sometimes be noted to protrude or herniate through the elastic areolar skin. This protrusion creates an odd step-off compared with the remainder of the smooth breast contour, and the sharp suture edge can often be plainly seen encircling the areolar border (**Fig. 7**). The underlying cause for this deformity relates to the laxity of the areolar skin that is then stented into a diameter that is too small, which allows the underlying breast parenchyma to protrude through. Treatment can involve one of 2 approaches. The easiest maneuver is to simply remove the interlocking suture. This approach allows the areola to expand and push back against the forces applied by the underlying breast parenchyma. The disadvantage of this approach is that the areola can then enlarge creating disproportion or asymmetry. A second treatment option is to revise the areola by incising a smaller areolar diameter. When the intervening skin between the new areola and the outer periareolar border is then

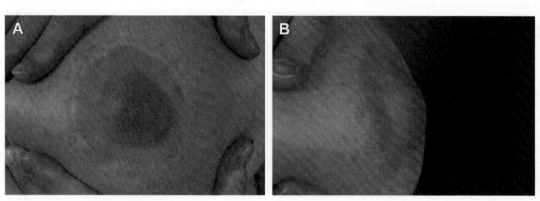

Fig. 7. (*A, B*) Areolar herniation.

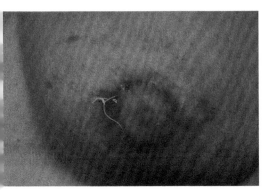

Fig. 8. Infected Teflon suture. The Teflon suture is exposed, and several small drainage holes can be seen along the periareolar incision.

de-epithelialized and a new interlocking suture applied, there will be enough tension on the areola to create a trampoline effect sufficient to hold the underlying breast parenchyma at bay and avoid any semblance of herniation. It is for this reason that the initial areolar diameters for a primary SPAIR are usually cut on the smaller side, ranging from 40 to 44 mm, in order to prevent subsequent areola herniation.

Infected Teflon suture

Although the Teflon suture affords numerous advantages related to long-term control of the periareolar opening as well as ease of use as it smoothly cinches down the periareolar opening, it does present as a persistent foreign body, and as such, in a small percentage of cases, the suture can become infected. Patients will present with a ring of redness around the areola often in association with small draining sinuses that may also expose the Teflon suture (**Fig. 8**). Although antibiotics targeted to routine skin flora are indicated, removal of the Teflon suture is the definitive treatment. With removal of the foreign body, the infection promptly clears. In many instances, sufficient scar will have developed such that the areola does not spread even despite the loss of support from the interlocking Teflon suture. However, postremoval spread of the areolar diameter will occur in most cases (**Fig. 9**). When this occurs, a simple redo of the periareolar closure with another Teflon suture well after the infection has settled will restore the desired periareolar size and shape (**Fig. 10**).

Rehypertrophy

In cases of rehypertrophy of the breast after SPAIR mammaplasty, simple reduction with liposuction followed by reapplication of the circumvertical pattern is a very effective management strategy. In this fashion, the blood supply to the NAC is only minimally disrupted, yet the volume reduction and the shape are easily managed with predictable and reliable results. During the circumvertical skin resection, only superficial skin removal is performed and deeper dissection into the breast is avoided. This technique preserves the blood supply to the NAC but yet allows the skin envelope to be retailored.

SUMMARY

Complications after the SPAIR mammaplasty are technique related and fortunately uncommon. With simple reapplication of the circumvertical skin pattern, most of these complications can be

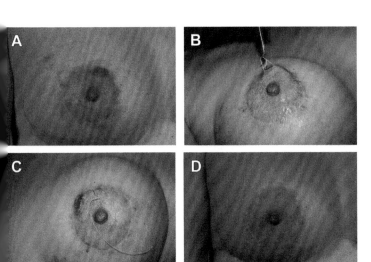

Fig. 9. (A) An infected Teflon suture often presents as a persistent nonhealing opening along the areolar incision. (B, C) The Teflon suture can be identified at the base of the wound and is easily removed. (D) With the removal of interlocking suture, wound healing rapidly occurs. However, with the loss of the suture support of the areolar opening, postoperative spreading of the areolar diameter can often occur.

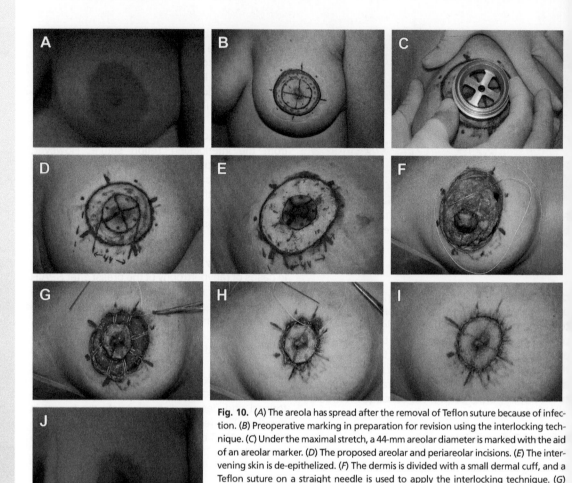

Fig. 10. (*A*) The areola has spread after the removal of Teflon suture because of infection. (*B*) Preoperative marking in preparation for revision using the interlocking technique. (*C*) Under the maximal stretch, a 44-mm areolar diameter is marked with the aid of an areolar marker. (*D*) The proposed areolar and periareolar incisions. (*E*) The intervening skin is de-epithelized. (*F*) The dermis is divided with a small dermal cuff, and a Teflon suture on a straight needle is used to apply the interlocking technique. (*G*) Appearance after placement of the interlocking suture. (*H*) Appearance after the interlocking suture is cinched down. (*I*) Final appearance. (*J*) Three-month postoperative appearance showing a reduced areolar diameter and an aesthetic periareolar scar.

predictably and reliably addressed. The SPAIR mammaplasty remains as an effective and versatile technique for breast reduction.

REFERENCES

1. American Society of Plastic Surgeons. 2014 Plastic surgery statistics. Available at: http://www.plasticsurgery.org/news/plastic-surgery-statistics/2014-statistics.html.

2. Hammond DC. Short scar periareolar inferior pedicle reduction (SPAIR) mammoplasty. Plast Reconstr Surg 1999;103(3):890–901.

3. Hammond DC, Alfonso D, Khuthaila DK. Mastopexy using the short scar periareolar inferior pedicle reduction technique. Plast Reconstr Surg 2008;212(5):1533–9.

4. Hammond D. Short scar periareolar inferior pedicle reduction (SPAIR) mammaplasty. Operat Tech Plast Reconstr Surg 1999;6:106.

5. Hammond D. Short scar periareolar inferior pedicle reduction (SPAIR) mammaplasty/mastopexy: how I do it step by step. Perspect Plast Surg 2001;15:67.

6. Hammond D. The SPAIR mammaplasty. Clin Plast Surg 2002;29:411.

7. Hammond D. The short scar periareolar inferior pedicle reduction (SPAIR) mammaplasty. Semin Plast Surg 2004;18:231 (New Trends in Reduction and Mastopexy).

8. WUuml;ringer E, Mader N, Posch E, et al. Nerve and vessel supplying ligamentous suspension of the mammary gland. Plast Reconstr Surg 1998;101: 1486–93.

9. Hammond DC, Khuthaila DK, Kim J. The interlocking Gore-Tex suture for control of areolar diameter and shape. Plast Reconstr Surg 2007; 119(3):804–9.

Management of Asymmetry After Breast Reduction

Onelio Garcia Jr, MD

KEYWORDS

- Breast asymmetry • Breast revision • Nipple malposition • Reduction mammaplasty complications

KEY POINTS

- Liposuction is an effective way to correct asymmetries of volume between the breast mounds. Ultrasound-assisted liposuction may be less traumatic.
- Implantation of an acellular dermal matrix or an absorbable mesh may be useful in cases where lower pole support is needed.
- Nipple malposition almost always involves high-riding nipples. Be mindful of the desired nipple position during the preoperative markings.
- A photograph grid is an effective way to assess preoperative and postoperative breast asymmetry.

INTRODUCTION

Reduction mammaplasty is currently the sixth most common surgical procedure performed on women by members of the American Society for Aesthetic Plastic Surgery. That same society reported 114,470 cases performed by its members in 2014.[1] Breast reduction surgery has achieved one of the highest patient satisfaction rates among plastic surgery procedures with 93% to 97% of patients indicating that they would undergo the procedure again.[2–5] The fact that this procedure enjoys tremendous success among patients despite reported complication rates of 53% is a testament to the efficacy of the operation in relieving the symptoms associated with macromastia and plastic surgeons becoming more adept at managing the more common postoperative problems associated with the surgery. Although complication rates reported in the literature range from 6% to 53%,[6–11] it is most likely that with careful scrutiny of postoperative results the overall complication rate for this operation will approximate the 43% figure quoted from the analysis of the BRAVO (Breast Reduction Assessment: Value and Outcome) study.[12] By far the most common complication reported in the literature is delayed wound healing followed by suture complications, hematoma, hypertrophic scars, nipple necrosis, fat necrosis, and seromas. Postoperative asymmetry is hardly ever mentioned in published series of breast reduction outcomes.

The possibility of postoperative breast asymmetry is always discussed with the patient as part of the preoperative informed consent process. Although it is currently the first complication listed in the breast reduction consent form created by the American Society of Plastic Surgeons, postoperative asymmetry requiring surgical revision is a rare event, occurring in less than 1% of cases. Currently, high-definition digital photography and standardized grids allow surgeons to critically assess their postoperative results (**Fig. 1**). Under these conditions the surgeon frequently notices minor asymmetries in nipple position, volume, or shape of the breasts; however, asymmetries noticeable enough for the patient to request revisionary surgery are a rare occurrence. Only one case of postoperative asymmetry was reported

Division of Plastic Surgery, University of Miami, Miller School of Medicine, 3850 Bird Road, Suite 102, Miami, FL 33146, USA
E-mail address: ogarciamd@aol.com

Clin Plastic Surg 43 (2016) 373–382
http://dx.doi.org/10.1016/j.cps.2015.12.002

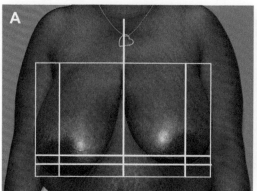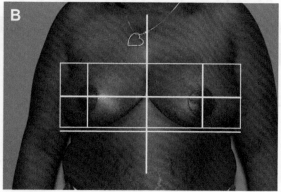

Fig. 1. (*A*) Preoperative evaluation of symmetry using grid patterns. (*B*) Postoperative evaluation (note the minor nipple asymmetry that is easily assessed with the grid pattern).

by the BRAVO study consisting of 179 patients. A review of my last 267 breast reductions revealed only two revisions related to postsurgical asymmetry, one for nipple asymmetry and the other for unilateral bottoming out phenomenon resulting in a noticeable shape asymmetry. After reviewing my cases I was convinced that the low revision rate for asymmetry was mostly caused by personally performing all my preoperative markings and the major portions of the operation on both breasts, consisting of the tissue resection and shaping. However, at our local plastic surgery training program at the University of Miami, School of Medicine, it is common for two surgeons to work simultaneously during a breast reduction. As in most plastic surgery training programs, it may be a resident in training working on one of the breasts. Even under these circumstances, significant postoperative breast asymmetry requiring revision remains a rare occurrence. In the past 3 years and more than 200 cases, there have not been any operations performed at that institution solely for the purpose of correcting post-breast-reduction asymmetry. This favorable experience is in contrast with a recent study reporting a 15% rate of significant asymmetry following vertical reduction mammaplasty.[13] Regardless of the technique used, appropriate preoperative markings and strict adherence to the markings during the surgery are still some of the most effective ways to prevent postmammaplasty asymmetry.

Breast asymmetry following reduction mammaplasty may involve the nipple-areolar complexes, differences in breast volume or shape, and/or location of the inframammary folds. Asymmetry that is noticeable early in the postoperative period is often the result of incorrect preoperative markings or poor surgical technique. Significant breast asymmetry may also occur years after a satisfactory initial result. Major weight fluctuations,

pregnancy, or the long-term effects of aging can contribute to late asymmetry. **Fig. 2** depict a 27-year-old woman who underwent bilateral reduction mammaplasty with acceptable early postoperative symmetry, then subsequently developed late stretch deformity of the lower poles (worse on the right side) resulting in noticeable asymmetry 2 years after her initial surgery.

ASYMMETRY OF THE NIPPLE-AREOLA COMPLEX

Malposition of the nipple-areola complex is a common occurrence following reduction mammaplasty. Most malpositions involve overelevation of the nipple-areola complex sometimes with asymmetry in relation to the contralateral side. A photometric study of 82 published reports of mastopexy and breast reduction reported a 41% incidence of nipple overelevation; however, none of the patients reviewed in the study had a nipple position below the level of maximum breast projection.[14]

Significant nipple-areola malposition is one of the most distressing complications for the post-breast-reduction patient. Several techniques have been described for lowering a high-riding nipple-areola. However, the revision surgery comes with the tradeoff of placing a scar in the upper pole of the breast above the areola, which some patients are unwilling to accept. Most of these techniques involve transposition of local flaps[15–17] or skin grafts.[18] Some authors have reported lowering the nipple-areola complex by inserting tissue expanders through periareolar incisions into the subcutaneous plane of the infraclavicular region to recruit upper pole skin and avoid visible scars on the superior breast surface.[19] In that series, the authors reported lowering the high-riding nipples by 2 cm to 6 cm

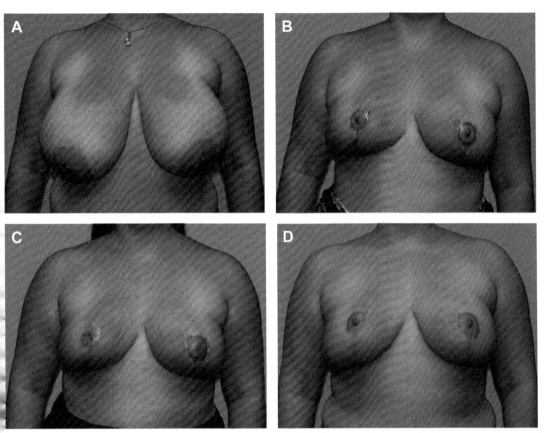

Fig. 2. (*A*) A 27 year old with macromastia and asymmetry. (*B*) Three weeks postreduction mammaplasty. (*C*) Two months postmammaplasty. (*D*) At 2 years postmammaplasty one can see recurrent ptosis and stretch deformity of the lower poles (worse on the *right* side) resulting in asymmetry.

without elastic tissue recoil following the expansion process. All the patients reported satisfaction with their nipple position after a 1- to 3-year follow-up period.

Recently Spear and coworkers[20] proposed a classification system for the evaluation of the high-riding nipple and an algorithm for surgical correction. The classification is based on the location of the nipple in relation to the vertical height of the breast as described by Malluci and Branford.[21] Nipple overelevation was defined as a location of less than 45% of the vertical breast height and three grades are described based on severity. Grade 1 (45%–35%) is considered mild, grade 2 (34%–25%) is considered moderate, and grade 3 (<25%) is considered severe. In addition, nipple malposition was also classified based on the relationship between the sternal notch, nipple-areola complex, and the inframammary fold. This further subclassified the nipple malposition into relative, absolute, or complex. Relative malposition is usually caused by a bottoming out deformity in which the nipple to inframammary fold distance is increased, making the

nipple appear high on the breast; however, the sternal notch to nipple distance is normal. In absolute malpositions the sternal notch to nipple distance is short and complex malpositions involve an element of both. In a subsequent letter to the editor, Swanson[22] questioned the reliability of this classification system on the basis that the anatomic landmarks used for the measurements are poorly defined and vary significantly from patient to patient. He proposes that the ideal nipple height should be defined as the apex or maximum projection point on the breast mound. However, Tebbets[23] reports that the ideal nipple location takes into account the relative base width of the breast and suggests the following formula for determining nipple location: base width of breast × 0.67 = desired nipple to inframammary fold distance. Some authors have suggested that elevation of the inframammary fold, placement of high-riding implants, and elliptical resection of lower pole skin may be viable options in some select patients not willing to accept breast scars above the superior border of the nipple-areola complex.

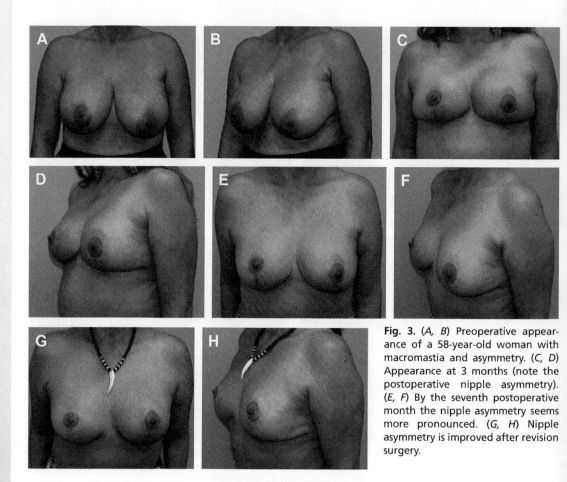

Fig. 3. (*A, B*) Preoperative appearance of a 58-year-old woman with macromastia and asymmetry. (*C, D*) Appearance at 3 months (note the postoperative nipple asymmetry). (*E, F*) By the seventh postoperative month the nipple asymmetry seems more pronounced. (*G, H*) Nipple asymmetry is improved after revision surgery.

A case of postreduction mammaplasty nipple asymmetry is presented. It involves a 58-year-old woman with macromastia and asymmetry of volume, shape, and nipple position (**Fig. 3**A, B). The photographs (**Fig. 3**C, D) depict the early postoperative result with residual asymmetry of the nipples. The asymmetry became more apparent as time went on (**Fig. 3**E, F) and revision surgery was performed at the patient's request. Results of the revision surgery are depicted (**Fig. 3**G, H).

The revision procedure consisted of reducing the left breast slightly using third-generation ultrasound-assisted liposuction to correct a minor volume discrepancy between the breasts. The nipple asymmetry was corrected by a revision mastopexy of the left breast (**Fig. 4**), raising the nipple-areola complex. The choice of the procedure took into account that the patient was unwilling to accept scars above the areola and was not bothered by the right nipple position, which I had determined was malpositioned slightly high on the breast mound. A detailed assessment of the correction is possible by examination of the prerevision and postrevision photographs on a grid pattern (**Fig. 5**).

Plastic surgeons may differ on their approach to this problem, but all can agree that successful management of nipple malposition with asymmetry is a complicated issue and that

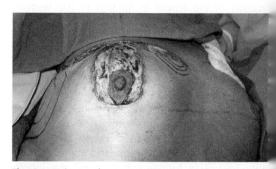

Fig. 4. A minor volume asymmetry was corrected with third-generation ultrasound-assisted liposuction of the left breast. The nipple asymmetry was corrected elevating the left nipple-areola complex by secondary mastopexy.

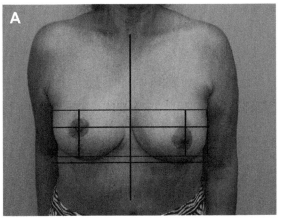 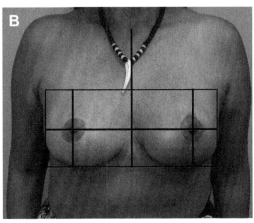

Fig. 5. (*A*) Postreduction mammaplasty nipple asymmetry. (*B*) Postrevision of the nipple asymmetry. The grid patterns allow detailed assessment of the results.

revisionary surgery comes with a price. Without a doubt, prevention is the best approach, particularly because a significant number of these complications are the result of poor preoperative planning or poor surgical execution and are avoidable.

Another type of asymmetry involving the nipple-areola complex is a differential in the postoperative circumference and/or geometric shape of the areolas. Although this may be caused by erroneous preoperative markings, areolar diameter differences are usually caused by skin tension differences between the breasts after wound closure. Correction of these complications is a more straightforward event than the correction of asymmetry caused by high-riding nipples.

It has been suggested that the ideal nipple/areola ratio is 3:1 and that an areolar diameter of 35 mm to 45 mm is considered attractive.[24] In any event areolar diameters of less than 50 mm are preferred by American women.[25] Using these parameters, most circumferential asymmetries can easily be corrected by applying the appropriate areolar marker circumference during the revision. When reducing or increasing areolar circumference, the area between the desired areola and the surrounding skin should be de-epithelialized to allow for a stronger wound closure. When the revision calls for decreasing the diameter of an abnormally wide areola, one should take into account the original causative factor, such as excessive tension, which can result in postrevision recurrence. Hammond[26–28] has suggested using an areolar closure technique in which he de-epithelializes the area between the desired areolar diameter and the surrounding skin creating a de-epithelialized dermal shelf that is closed by a buried purse-string Gortex suture. Using this technique he has been successful in equalizing the

tension around the areola and maintaining the desired diameter long term in hundreds of patients.

An ovoid or inverted teardrop areolar shape is a common occurrence following the use of a mosque-dome (LeJour) or keyhole (Wise) marking patterns for breast reduction. When the deformity appears unilaterally resulting in a shape difference between the areolas it becomes more noticeable and distressing to the patient. Swanson's[14] photometric study involving 82 published reports of mastopexy and breast reduction reported an 84% incidence of the deformity following these preoperative marking patterns. He suggests complete closure of the skin in the desired areolar location leaving the nipple-areola complex beneath the closure and then bringing out the nipple-areola through a circular opening of the desired dimensions. This equalizes the tension around the areola and maintains a circular shape. At the very least, applying an areolar marker of the desired dimensions around the areolar closure when using keyhole or mosque-dome patterns and closing it accordingly during the initial surgery prevents the deformity in most cases.

ASYMMETRIES OF BREAST MOUND VOLUME AND SHAPE

Significant asymmetry involving the breast mounds is particularly distressing to patients because of its interference with wearing standard brassieres and certain feminine garments. Asymmetry is noticeable during the preoperative examination in a significant number of patients with macromastia. When the asymmetry of volume is significant, many patients seem as distressed about that problem as they are about the symptoms related to their breast hypertrophy. In these cases the goal of reduction mammaplasty is not only to reduce the breast volume and improve the shape but also to correct the asymmetry. Unfortunately, despite best efforts, critical evaluation of reduction mammaplasty patients reveals that asymmetries occur postoperatively in most cases. Fortunately most of these are minor asymmetries that are of no consequence to the patient and are only appreciated by careful scrutiny of the postoperative photographs.

Occasionally the postreduction mammaplasty asymmetry is so severe that the patient requests revisionary surgery. When revisions of the breast mounds do occur, it is frequently for correction of the bottoming out phenomenon in which the breast parenchyma descends below the inframammary fold with stretching of the inferior pole skin, increasing the nipple to inframammary fold distance. When the deformity occurs unilaterally, it can result in significant postoperative breast asymmetry. This situation is usually a consequence of disruption of the inframammary fold attachments and/or leaving too much parenchymal tissue inferiorly during the original surgery. There are several approaches for the correction of the bottoming out deformity; however, they should be individualized to correct the causative factor. When the deformity is created by inadequate resection of the inferior pole parenchyma, Hall-Findlay[29] suggests further resection of the inferior parenchyma without repositioning of the inframammary fold or skin resection. Hammond,[30] however, prefers to correct the deformity with a vertical scar revision, plicating any excess skin along the vertical closure. Both of these authors, however, perform vertical mammaplasty procedures that seldom violate the inframammary fold attachments.

The surgical correction of bottoming out deformities following inverted-T mammaplasty procedures often needs to include reattachment of the inframammary fold to the chest wall. Occasionally, implanting a sheet of acellular dermal matrix or an absorbable mesh is helpful in reinforcing the fold and/or providing lower pole support. Use of these products can help avoid recurrences in large breasts or in patients with attenuated tissues.

All reduction mammaplasty techniques have the potential for postoperative volume asymmetries. This is particularly true in patients with significant preoperative asymmetry or cases with high-volume resections. Seldom is the asymmetry severe enough that it prevents the patient from wearing a standard brassiere because there is more than a cup size differential between the breasts. The incidence of revisionary surgery for the sole purpose of correcting breast mound volume discrepancies is fortunately rare. Several authors have proposed breast liposuction as a method of breast reduction alone or in combination with open mammaplasty procedures.[31–33] Volume extraction by liposuction is a safe and efficient method to correct the asymmetry in cases where the discrepancy involves only a volume differential between the breasts. Several authors have reported using ultrasound-assisted lipoplasty for volume removal in the breast with good outcomes and low complication rates.[34,35] I frequently perform third-generation pulsed, solid probe ultrasound-assisted liposuction to reduce breast volume and have found it to be highly effective.

Rarely open procedures may be necessary to correct breast mound volume asymmetries particularly in cases where recurrent ptosis is also being corrected. There is some controversy about the approach to repeat reduction mammaplasty.

Some authors suggest strict adherence to the original dermoglandular pedicle supporting the nipple-areola complex.[36] The University of Michigan reported their 12-year experience with repeat reduction mammaplasty and found a 37% major complication rate.[37] Knowledge of the type of dermoglandular pedicle used during the initial operation was not helpful in this series. Inferior pedicles were associated with the highest complication rates even when the secondary surgery used the same type of pedicle. Revisions that resorted to a free nipple areola graft were not associated with any major complications and the authors recommend this approach for revision mammaplasty surgery. Other authors believe that knowledge of the pedicle technique used in the initial surgery does not affect outcomes in secondary reduction mammaplasty.[38] The University of Rochester reported their experience with secondary reduction mammaplasty and concluded that the procedure was a safe and viable option when performed with either a similar or a different technique than the initial mammaplasty.[39] Although primary reduction mammaplasty is a common procedure in most major plastic surgery training programs, it is interesting that only 10 cases of secondary reductions were identified at this institution over a 37-year period and only one of the cases was performed solely for correction of volume asymmetry.

A case of late-onset severe breast asymmetry secondary to unilateral bottoming out deformity is presented. A 64-year-old woman with severe macromastia is depicted in **Fig. 6**A, B. The photographs in **Fig. 6**C, D correspond to 3 weeks postreduction mammaplasty using an inferior pedicle technique and inverted-T-type incisions. At 4 months postsurgery, note that the left inframammary fold is still attached (**Fig. 6**E, F). At 14 months there is some loss of definition of the left inframammary fold (**Fig. 6**G, H). On the 2-year postoperative visit there is total loss of definition of the left inframammary fold and the unsupported breast has descended

inferiorly into the left upper abdomen (**Fig. 6**I, J). The patient subsequently underwent revision surgery, which consisted of reattachment of the left inframammary fold reinforced with an 8 cm × 16 cm sheet of AlloMax (Bard-Davol, Warwick, RI) acellular dermal matrix attached to the chest wall (**Fig. 7**). The 1-year postrevision photographs are depicted in **Fig. 6**K, L. The left inframammary fold is reestablished (**Fig. 8**A, B) and the breast shape is restored.

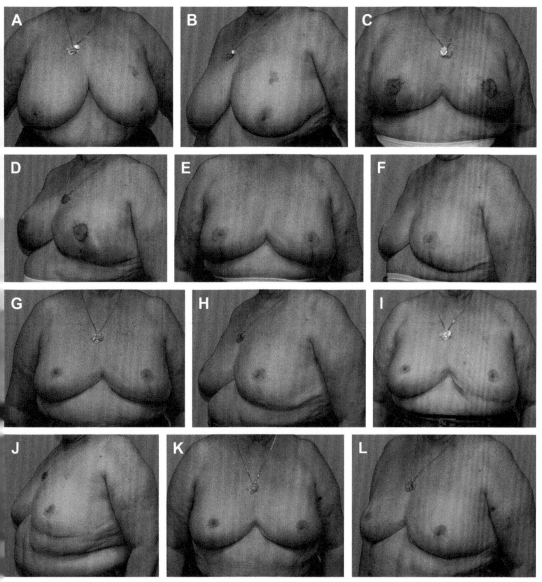

Fig. 6. (*A, B*) A 64-year-old woman with severe macromastia. (*C, D*) Appearance 3 weeks after reduction mammaplasty with an inferior pedicle technique. (*E, F*) Appearance at 4 months with a well-defined left inframammary fold. (*G, H*) At 14 months there is some loss of definition of the left inframammary fold. (*I, J*) Two years after the surgery there is loss of support of the left breast with bottoming out resulting in severe breast asymmetry. (*K, L*) Appearance 1 year after revision of the left breast for correction of the asymmetry.

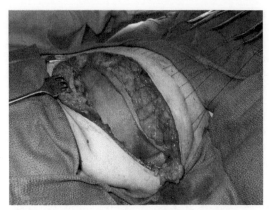

Fig. 7. The left inframammary fold was reinforced with implantation of an acellular dermal matrix.

DISCUSSION

Although reduction mammaplasty is associated with a high complication rate, most of the complications encountered are usually minor and related to wound healing. Revision surgery to address these problems is common and usually consists of scar revisions. Postoperative breast asymmetry of a mild degree is also common. A detailed assessment of post-breast-reduction photographs undoubtedly reveals asymmetries in most cases. Fortunately most of these are so minor that the patient hardly notices them if at all. Asymmetry after a breast reduction severe enough to warrant revision is a rare occurrence.

When severe asymmetries occur, the approach to revision surgery needs to be individualized depending on the problem. For example, the asymmetry could be the result of nipple malposition or it could consist of a volume or shape discrepancy between the breast mounds, two problems requiring very different corrective measures. Some of the techniques involved in secondary breast revision surgery may be more complex than the original operation and require careful, detailed preoperative planning. Do not hesitate to use a dermal matrix or an absorbable mesh when reinforcement or support is needed. As with any secondary revision surgery, the surgeon should take every step necessary to avoid having to revise the revision. Surgery to correct high-riding nipples causing asymmetry may place scars in conspicuous areas high in the breast mound. Discuss with the patient the tradeoffs of the revision and make sure that the nipple asymmetry is severe enough to warrant the procedure.

Currently reduction mammaplasty is associated with high patient satisfaction rates because the procedure is highly effective in reducing the symptoms associated with macromastia while creating an aesthetically pleasing breast shape. Regarding postmammaplasty asymmetry, Elizabeth Hall-Findlay commented; "it is interesting that the patients who seem most bothered by the asymmetry are the ones who were asymmetric before surgery." I agree wholeheartedly.

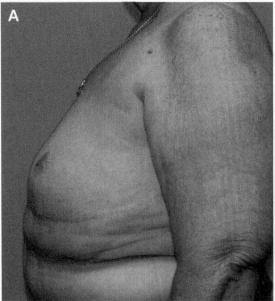
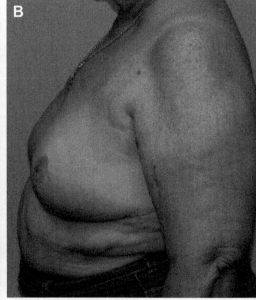

Fig. 8. (*A*) Pre-revision deformity of left inframammary fold. (*B*) At 1 year after re-establishment of the left inframammary fold and restoration of breast shape.

REFERENCES

1. American Society for Aesthetic Plastic Surgery, Cosmetic Surgery National Data Bank Statistics, 2014.

2. Schnur PL, Schnur DP, Petty PM, et al. Reduction mammoplasty: an outcome study. Plast Reconstr Surg 1997;100:875.

3. Nahai FR, Nahai F. MOC-PSSM CME article: breast reduction. Plast Reconstr Surg 2008;121:1.

4. Davis GM, Ringler SL, Short K, et al. Reduction mammoplasty: long term efficacy, morbidity, and patient satisfaction. Plast Reconstr Surg 1995;96: 1106.

5. Hughes LA, Mahoney JL. Patient satisfaction with reduction mammoplasty: an early survey. Aesthetic Plast Surg 1993;17:345.

6. Dabbah A, Lehman JA, Parker MG, et al. Reduction mammaplasty: an outcome analysis. Ann Plast Surg 1995;35:337.

7. Economides NG, Sifakis F. Reduction mammoplasty: a study of sequelae. Breast J 1997;3:69.

8. Lista F, Ahmad J. Vertical scar reduction mammoplasty: a 15 year experience including a review of 250 consecutive cases. Plast Reconstr Surg 2006; 117:2152.

9. Miller BJ, Morris SF, Sigurdson LL. Prospective study of outcomes after reduction mammoplasty. Plast Reconstr Surg 2005;115:1025.

10. Lejour M. Vertical mammoplasty: early complications after 250 personal consecutive cases. Plast Reconstr Surg 1999;104:764.

11. Collins ED, Kerrigan CL, Kim M, et al. The effectiveness of surgical and non-surgical interventions in relieving the symptoms of macromastia. Plast Reconstr Surg 2002;109:1556.

12. Cunningham BL, Gear AJL, Kerrigan CL, et al. Analysis of breast reduction complications derived from the BRAVO study. Plast Reconstr Surg 2005;115: 1597.

13. Adham M, Sawan K, Lovelace C, et al. Unfavorable outcomes with vertical breast reduction mammoplasty: part II. Aesthet Surg J 2011;31:40.

14. Swanson E. A retrospective photometric study of 82 published reports of mastopexy and breast reduction. Plast Reconstr Surg 2011;128:1282.

15. Frenkiel BA, Pacifico MD, Ritz M, et al. A solution to the high riding nipple-areola complex. Aesthetic Plast Surg 2010;34:525.

16. Mohmand H, Nassan A. Double U-plasty for correction of geometric malposition of the nipple-areola complex. Plast Reconstr Surg 2002;109:2019.

17. Elsahy NI. Correction of abnormally high nipples after reduction mammoplasty. Aesthetic Plast Surg 1990;14:21.

18. Spear SL, Hoffman S. Relocation of the displaced nipple-areola by reciprocal skin grafts. Plast Reconstr Surg 1998;101:1355.

19. Colwell AS, May JW, Slavin SA. Lowering the postoperative high riding nipple. Plast Reconstr Surg 2007;120:596.

20. Spear SL, Albino FP, Al-Attar A. Classification and management of the postoperative high-riding nipple. Plast Reconstr Surg 2013;131:1413.

21. Malluci P, Branford OA. Concepts in aesthetic breast dimensions: analysis of the ideal breast. J Plast Reconstr Aesthet Surg 2012;65:8.

22. Swanson E. Letter to the editor. Defining nipple displacement and the prevention and treatment of the high-riding nipple. Plast Reconstr Surg 2014; 133:64e.

23. Tebbets JB. A process for quantifying aesthetic and functional breast surgery: I. Quantifying optimal nipple position and vertical and horizontal skin excess for mastopexy and breast reduction. Plast Reconstr Surg 2013;132:65.

24. Bostwick J III. Applied aesthetics. In: Bostwick J III, editor. Plastic and reconstructive breast surgery. 2nd edition. St Louis (MO): Quality Medical; 2000. p. 125–57.

25. Swanson E. A measurement system for evaluation of shape changes and proportions after cosmetic breast surgery. Plast Reconstr Surg 2012;129:982.

26. Hammond DC. The SPAIR mammoplasty. Clin Plast Surg 2002;29:411.

27. Hammond DC. Short scar periareolar inferior pedicle reduction (SPAIR) mammoplasty: operative techniques. Plast Reconstr Surg 1999;6:106.

28. Hammond DC. Short scar periareolar inferior pedicle reduction (SPAIR) mammoplasty/mastopexy: how I do it step by step. Perspect Plast Surg 2001;15:61.

29. Hall-Findlay EJ. Vertical breast reduction using the superomedial pedicle. In: Spear SL, Willey SC, Robb GL, et al, editors. Surgery of the breast: principles and art. 3rd edition. Philadelphia: Lippincott Williams and Wilkins; 2011. p. 1045–62.

30. Hammond DC. Short periareolar inferior pedicle reduction mammoplasty. In: Spear SL, Willey SC, Robb GL, et al, editors. Surgery of the breast: principles and art. 3rd edition. Philadelphia: Lippincott Williams and Wilkins; 2011. p. 1063–77.

31. Moskowitz MJ, Muskin E, Baxt A. Outcome study in liposuction breast reduction. Plast Reconstr Surg 2004;114:55.

32. LeJour M. Vertical mammaplasty and liposuction of the breast. Plast Reconstr Surg 1994;94:100.

33. Akyurek M. Contouring the inferior pole of the breast in vertical mammaplasty: suction assisted lipectomy versus direct defatting. Plast Reconstr Surg 2011; 127:1314.

34. Di Giuseppe A. Breast reduction with ultrasound-assisted lipoplasty. Plast Reconstr Surg 2003;112:71.

35. Goes JC, Landecker A. Ultrasound–assisted lipo-plasty (UAL) in breast surgery. Aesthetic Plast Surg 2002;26:1.

36. Hudson DA, Skoll PJ. Repeat reduction mamma-plasty. Plast Reconstr Surg 1999;104:401.

37. Patel SP, Brown DL, Cederna PS. Repeat bilateral reduction mammaplasty: a 12-year experience. Plast Reconstr Surg 2010;126:263.

38. Ahmad J, McIsaac SM, Lista F. Does knowledge of the initial technique affect outcomes after repeated breast reduction? Plast Reconstr Surg 2012;129:11.

39. Losee JE, Caldwell EH, Serletti JM. Secondary reduction mammaplasty: is using a different pedicle safe? Plast Reconstr Surg 2000; 106:1004.

Management of Recurrent or Persistent Macromastia

Ryan E. Austin, MD[a], Frank Lista, MD, FRCSC[b], Jamil Ahmad, MD, FRCSC[b],*

KEYWORDS

- Breast reduction • Complication • Mammary hypertrophy • Recurrent • Reduction mammaplasty
- Vertical scar • Revision • Pedicle

KEY POINTS

- Repeated breast reduction can be a safe and reliable procedure, even in cases of unknown initial pedicle, with little risk of vascular compromise of the nipple-areola complex (NAC).
- It is important to determine whether the NAC is adequately positioned, because this determines whether transposition of the NAC is required in addition to the inferior wedge resection and liposuction used for volume reduction.
- Liposuction is a useful adjunct in repeated breast reduction, because it allows for volume reduction while at the same time minimizing damage to the blood supply of the breast NAC.
- It is important to rule out malignancy as a potential cause of recurrent macromastia, particularly if the recurrence is unilateral.

INTRODUCTION

Breast reduction continues to be one of the most commonly performed procedures in plastic surgery, with more than 114,000 breast reductions performed in 2014, according to the American Society for Aesthetic Plastic Surgery.[1]

Recurrent macromastia can be defined as the accumulation of excessive breast tissue after breast reduction. Excess breast tissue is a function of 2 factors: (1) the amount of excess tissue in the breast and (2) the location of excess tissue in the breast. Persistent macromastia describes continued breast tissue excess despite previous breast reduction.

Repeated breast reduction goes by several other names in the literature, including secondary breast reduction and revision breast reduction. All of these terms refer to volume reduction procedures after primary breast reduction. For the remainder of this article, the technique is referred to as repeated breast reduction. This article on the management of recurrent or persistent macromastia reviews key principles for repeated breast reduction and the authors' approach to this potentially difficult problem.

BACKGROUND

Despite reduction mammaplasty being one of the most commonly performed procedures in plastic surgery,[1] the literature on outcomes after repeated breast reduction is limited to a handful of case series[2–4] and case studies.[5–9] Unfortunately, the sparse literature that does exist presents conflicting opinions and approaches to repeated breast reduction. Some investigators report significant complications in repeated breast reduction cases, including complete loss of the NAC,[6,8] and advise that repeated breast reduction be approached

Disclosures: The authors declared no potential conflicts of interest with respect to the authorship and publication of this article. There are no sources of financial support to disclose regarding this article.
^a Division of Plastic and Reconstructive Surgery, University of Toronto, 149 College Street, 5th Floor, Suite 508, Toronto, Ontario M5T 1P5, Canada; ^b Division of Plastic and Reconstructive Surgery, University of Toronto, Toronto, Ontario, Canada
* Corresponding author.
E-mail address: drahmad@theplasticsurgeryclinic.com

Clin Plastic Surg 43 (2016) 383–393
http://dx.doi.org/10.1016/j.cps.2015.12.004
0094-1298/16/$ – see front matter © 2016 Elsevier Inc. All rights reserved.

with great apprehension.[6,8,10,11] Some investigators even advocate liberal use of free nipple grafting in these cases.[6,8,10,12] Meanwhile, other investigators have reported good results and believe repeated breast reduction can be a safe option, even in cases where the original mammaplasty technique is unknown.[5,7,9,13]

A review of the case series published in the literature reports 88 patients having undergone repeated breast reduction, with 75 of these patients requiring transposition of the NAC (**Table 1**). Lejour[5] reported good results after vertical mammaplasty in 14 patients with no complications. She noted that liposuction was a safe technique that allowed for volume reduction without compromising vascularity to the NAC.

Hudson and Skoll[6] reviewed 16 repeated breast reduction patients, of which 8 required NAC transposition. Three patients in this cohort suffered vascular compromise of the NAC, with 2 leading to complete unilateral loss. Among these 3 cases, 2 occurred in the setting of a new dermoglandular pedicle (primary superomedial pedicle revised to inferior pedicle; primary inferior pedicle revised to superior pedicle) whereas the other occurred in the repeated use of an inferior pedicle. They suggested using the same pedicle, if known, when the NAC required transposition and otherwise free nipple grafting if the initial pedicle was unknown.

Losee and colleagues[7] reported on 10 patients undergoing repeated breast reduction. A different technique/pedicle was used in 7 of the 10 cases, although only 3 cases involved complete transection of the previous pedicle.[10] Five minor complications were reported in 3 patients, with no cases of NAC vascular compromise. Their group concluded that repeated breast reduction is a safe option when using either a similar or different technique.

Patel and colleagues[8] reported a major complication rate of 37.5% in 8 patients undergoing repeated breast reduction. Furthermore, the investigators reported a 100% complication rate among the 3 patients where an inferior pedicle was used for both the primary and secondary procedure, including 1 case of NAC necrosis. They suggested that free nipple grafting might be the technique of choice for repeated breast reduction as there were no complications in the 2 cases included in their series.

Sultan and colleagues[9] reported on 15 patients who underwent repeated breast reduction using a vertical scar with superior or superomedial pedicle after primary inverted T scar breast reduction. The initial pedicle was known in only 4 of the cases and all 4 were inferior pedicles. They reported 1 complication of unilateral NAC epidermolysis, which healed fully with conservative management. They concluded that this approach is safe and provides good aesthetic results.

A review of the literature reveals 20 documented complications among the 88 patients reported to have undergone repeated breast reduction. The majority of the complications (14 of 20) would be classified as minor complications (ie, delayed wound healing, scarring, and recurrent asymmetry) with only 3 patients experiencing complete NAC necrosis[6,8] and 2 patients experiencing of

Table 1
Complications reported from case series of patients undergoing repeated breast reduction

	No. of Patients (No. of Breasts)	No. of Complications	Nature of Complications
Lejour,[5] 1997	14 (28)	0	N/A
Hudson & Skoll,[6] 1999	16 (28)	8	NAC necrosis (2) NAC compromise (1) Scar/dog ear (2) Wound-healing complications (2) Hematoma (1)
Losee et al,[7] 2000	10 (?)	5	Delayed wound healing (3) Delayed nipple sensation return (2)
Patel et al,[8] 2010	8 (16)	3	NAC necrosis (1) Seroma (1) Abscess (1)
Ahmad et al,[13] 2012	25 (48)	3	Recurrent asymmetry (2) Cellulitis (1)
Sultan et al,[9] 2013	15 (28)	1	NAC epidermolysis (1)

NAC vascular compromise or epidermolysis.[6,9] In all 3 reported cases of total NAC necrosis, an inferior pedicle was used for the revision procedure after either a primary inferior pedicle (2 cases) or a primary superomedial pedicle (1 case).

In 2012, the authors reported experience with repeated breast reduction in 25 patients using a modified technique for vertical scar reduction mammaplasty[13]; 21 patients required transposition of the NAC, and in approximately half of the cases the initial pedicle was unknown. Overall, 3 patients experienced minor complications; however, there were no cases of either partial or total NAC necrosis. The authors concluded that the use of vertical scar reduction mammaplasty with liposuction for repeated breast reduction is safe, even when the initial pedicle is unknown. Since this initial report, the authors have performed repeated breast reduction on more than 40 patients.[14] To date, there have been no documented cases of either partial or total nipple necrosis using the authors' modified technique for repeated breast reduction. Additionally, there have been no significant issues with skin necrosis or clinically detectable fat necrosis, which can also occur due to compromised blood supply during repeated breast reduction.

ETIOLOGY

When discussing the etiology of recurrent or persistent macromastia, it is important to elucidate the precise nature of a patient's concerns. Patients presenting with macromastia despite previous breast reduction may be frustrated, having already invested time, energy, and money into a primary surgical procedure that did not meet their expectations. In any patient presenting with macromastia after previous breast reduction, it is important to clarify whether there has been any change in the size or shape of the breasts since the procedure as well as what those changes were and when they occurred. This information is critical in determining the cause of the breast volume excess.

Recurrent or persistent macromastia should be considered a problem of (1) inadequate volume reduction during the primary operation, (2) inadequate breast shape, or (3) breast tissue hypertrophy. Although only breast tissue hypertrophy represents true recurrent macromastia, it is important to consider these other etiologies when assessing a patient for repeated breast reduction because these help define the goals of surgery.

Inadequate Primary Volume Reduction

Inadequate volume reduction during the primary breast reduction is a frequent indication for repeated breast reduction. This may be due to technical factors but also may be related to a patient's goals and expectations of the procedure. Although it is important to understand patients' goals, it is equally important to manage their expectations preoperatively and ensure that they have a clear understanding the limitations of breast reduction surgery.

Patients often discuss desired postoperative breast size in relation to brassiere cup size. In 1984, Regnault and Daniel[15] described an algorithm predicting the amount of tissue resection required to change the bra cup size based on chest circumference.[12] Since then, several methods for predicting the resection amount in a reduction mammaplasty have been described, using either direct measurements[16–18] or 3-D surface imaging.[19] The authors, however, do not find these methods applicable or reliable, particularly given the lack of standardization between bra manufacturers.[20]

Although it is helpful to ask patients preoperatively about their desired postoperative breast size, more importantly, it is more important to elucidate whether they prefer to be on the smaller or larger end of that range. Not only does this involve patients into the decision making process, it also helps determine how extensive a planned resection should be.

Inadequate Breast Shape

Pseudoptosis, or bottoming-out, was originally defined by Regnault[21] as a breast shape where the gland descends inferior to the inframammary crease but the nipple remains above the crease. For patients who have just undergone a reduction mammaplasty to reduce and reshape the breast only to see this shape lost over time, pseudoptosis can be a significant concern. Pseudoptosis can also, in turn, make the NAC appear superiorly malpositioned. Although not true recurrent macromastia, because pseudoptosis represents a change in breast shape not an increase in breast volume, patients may not recognize or understand this difference.

To understand how this deformity may be prevented and corrected, an understanding of why it occurs is needed. Pseudoptosis can be thought of a failure of parenchymal support and skin support due to the excess weight of breast tissue. This failure may occur naturally with age, because the dermis naturally thins and loses elasticity, or it may occur after a primary reduction mammaplasty. Postoperative pseudoptosis is a commonly recognized deformity after inverted T scar/inferior pedicle breast reductions.[22–24] Conceptually this makes sense, because the procedure relies on the skin to support the breast while leaving the weight of the breast in the inferior pole as the inferior pedicle. On the other hand, vertical scar/superior or superomedial pedicle breast reductions use parenchymal supporting sutures to cone the breast, removing the deforming weight of the inferior pole of the breast.[25]

Studies looking at the 3-D shape of the breast over time following breast reduction demonstrate that shape changes in the breast occur over the first postoperative year with little change occurring thereafter, suggesting that pseudoptosis may be a relatively early postoperative occurrence.[26–28]

It is important to recognize the difference between pseudoptosis and true ptosis. In cases of pseudoptosis the NAC is, by definition, in an acceptable position. Therefore, significant risk can be avoided by not attempting to reposition the NAC in these cases.

Another common problem after breast reduction can be asymmetry. Asymmetry is common in breast surgery and all patients have some degree of preoperative asymmetry, whether they realize it or not. It is important to point out these asymmetries to patients prior to surgery.

In some cases, the area of concern after breast reduction is the lateral chest wall as opposed to the breast. For patients, the transition between the lateral breast and lateral chest wall is poorly defined due to fatty fullness of the lateral chest compartment.[29] In these patients, breast size and shape after breast reduction may be adequate whereas their concern is really with contour of the lateral chest wall. Liposuction and, in some cases, excision of the redundant skin may be indicated as opposed to repeated breast reduction.

Breast Tissue Hypertrophy

True recurrent macromastia, or the redevelopment of breast hypertrophy after breast reduction, is fortunately a rare occurrence. Although attempts have been made to define breast hypertrophy by breast volume or bra cup size,[30] the authors suggest it is important not to attempt to correlate a patient's breast size or body mass index with subjective symptoms. Studies have found no direct correlation between preoperative breast size, the severity of preoperative symptoms, and the postoperative degree of improvement of symptoms.[31,32] Recurrent macromastia can be thought of as the development of breast enlargement after breast reduction, such that the patient experiences a significant impact on their functional symptoms and/or their aesthetic outcome. Not

only does this remove all weight and size parameters from the definition of recurrent macromastia but also it provides a more person-centered definition of the condition.[33]

There are several possible causes for recurrent macromastia, including weight gain and hormonal changes (eg, pregnancy and lactation).[3,9,24,34] An important potential cause of recurrent macromastia that must never be overlooked is a neoplastic process in the breast, particularly if the recurrence is unilateral.

One unique cause of recurrent macromastia is juvenile hypertrophy of the breast, also referred to in the literature as virginal hypertrophy, juvenile macromastia, or juvenile gigantomastia.[35,36] Representing approximately 2% of all breast pathology in adolescents,[37] juvenile hypertrophy is characterized by a diffuse enlargement of the breast without the presence of a distinct mass or nodularity.[35,38] Adolescents with this condition often suffer from significant functional and psychological distress, and the severity of these symptoms often necessitates surgical intervention prior to the end of puberty, which may contribute to the high recurrence rate.[36] Although a full discussion of the management of juvenile hypertrophy of the breast is beyond the scope of this article, this is an important diagnosis to be aware of and to warn adolescent patients about prior to primary reduction mammaplasty.

PREOPERATIVE CONSIDERATIONS
History and Physical Examination

Women presenting with recurrent or persistent macromastia range greatly in age, breast size, and body habitus. The goals of these patients also vary greatly, ranging from purely for symptom relief to purely aesthetic, with most on a spectrum somewhere between the two.

The functional assessment for these patients begins with a thorough review of the symptoms they have as a result of their macromastia. Kerrigan and colleagues[30] identified 7 symptoms specific to breast hypertrophy (upper back pain, neck pain, shoulder pain, arm pain, arm numbness, rashes, and bra strap grooving) and found greater postoperative improvement in women reporting at least 2 of 7 physical symptoms all/most of the time. Although the authors find it helpful to review these symptoms with patients to determine their functional status, it is equally important to clarify which symptoms were present prior to their primary reduction mammaplasty and to what degree they changed after surgery.

The aesthetic assessment for these patients focuses on the size and shape changes of the breast since the primary breast reduction procedure. A patient with recurrent or persistent macromastia may be more bothered by breast shape or spreading of their scars than the actual size of the breasts, and this is important to clarify and discuss. The patient should describe what changes they have noticed in the size and shape of the breast, whether these changes have been symmetric, and over what time period these changes have occurred.

In patients with recurrent macromastia, it is important to assess for possible systemic causes. Patients should be asked about changes in their general health, weight changes, and if they have been pregnant and/or have breastfed since their previous surgery, because all these factors could contribute to changes in breast size. Although studies have demonstrated a decreased risk of breast cancer after breast reduction,[39–42] patients presenting with recurrent macromastia should be asked about changes in the breast that may be concerning for breast cancer, including new lumps/masses, nipple discharge, and skin changes, as well as the timing and results of their most recent mammogram.

A thorough physical examination is important in the assessment of any patient presenting with recurrent or persistent macromastia. All patients should have their height and weight recorded at the time of presentation. The clinician should then perform a thorough breast examination, with a focus on skin and scar quality as well as breast size and shape. Any asymmetry between the breasts should be noted. Careful attention should be paid to the areas of excess glandular tissue and the presence of ptosis versus pseudoptosis. Finally, a screening breast examination should be performed, palpating the breasts for any abnormal masses.

Although little evidence exists regarding specific risk factors associated with repeated breast reduction, there is ample evidence regarding risk factors for primary breast reduction. As a result, the authors do not perform this procedure on active smokers due to the well-documented risks of smokers undergoing breast reduction, particularly regarding delayed wound healing and wound infection.[43–47] Patients presenting for repeated breast reduction who are active smokers are instructed to quit smoking for at least 4 weeks preoperatively and 4 weeks postoperatively to decrease their risk of complications.[48,49]

Previous Operative Records

All efforts should be made to obtain the surgical reports from the previous surgery; however, these records are often unobtainable. Even when the operative records are available, they may not contain enough detail to be of any use.

Informed Consent

It is important to have a thorough and well-documented discussion about the potential risks associated with repeated breast reduction. Although the authors believe this is a safe and effective procedure, the risk of complications is always a concern in revision surgery. **Table 2** outlines the common and significant risks that can occur during repeated breast reduction.

TIMING OF REPEATED BREAST REDUCTION

The shape of the breast can change significantly in the early postoperative period. Studies have shown that the postoperative volume of the breast decrease in the range of 8% to 14% during the first 3 months postoperatively with the resolution of edema.[27,50] Studies examining changes in 3-D morphology of the breast after breast reduction show that breast shape stabilizes 6 to 9 months after surgery, with little change beyond 1 year.[26,28,50] It is important to ensure that sufficient time has passed for all swelling to resolve and for the breast to assume a stable aesthetic result prior to attempting revision surgery. During this time, some patients may actually become less bothered by small degrees of asymmetry and further surgery may be avoided.

Additionally, use of the authors' modified technique is predicated on the assumption that the NAC has been revascularized by the surrounding

Table 2	
Complications after repeated breast reduction surgery	
Early Complications	**Late Complications**
Bleeding/hematoma	Over-resection/under-resection
Seroma	Asymmetry
Infection (cellulitis, abscess)	Contour irregularities
Wound dehiscence	Pseudoptosis
Fat necrosis	Hypertrophic scar
NAC vascular compromise/necrosis	NAC malposition/ shape
Skin vascular compromise/necrosis	NAC widening
Altered nipple sensation	Permanent suture infection/extrusion
—	Inability to lactate

tissues, allowing for adequate blood supply of the NAC if the initial pedicle happens to be divided during repeated breast reduction. Although the authors cannot say what the minimal or optimal time interval should be before repeated breast reduction to increase the safety of the procedure and reduce the risk of complications, their approach has been to wait at least 1 year postoperatively before performing any major revision procedures after breast reduction.

OPERATIVE TECHNIQUE

The authors exclusively perform their modified technique for vertical scar reduction mammaplasty for all patients presenting for repeated breast reduction (**Figs. 1** and **2**). This technique allows for resection of breast tissue while maintaining an adequate blood supply to the NAC and remaining breast tissue. It has proved safe in cases of repeated breast reduction where a different skin resection pattern was used (ie, inverted T scar) and/or a different pedicle was used during the initial breast reduction. To date, the authors have used this technique on more than 40 patients and have not experienced any cases of NAC necrosis.

Understanding the Blood Supply of the Nipple-Areola Complex

Understanding the blood supply of the breast and the NAC is of particular importance in repeated breast reduction given the concern of NAC necrosis. Anatomic[51,52] and imaging[53] studies have shown that the primary blood supply to the breast comes from the medial aspect and is supplied by perforators from the internal mammary artery. Work by le Roux and colleagues[54,55] has shown that the venous drainage of the NAC is through an extensive superficial plexus. It is important in cases of repeated breast reduction to preserve as much of the arterial and venous supply as possible.

One specific concern in repeated breast reduction is transection of the previous pedicle for cases in which a new pedicle is selected. Evidence from recent studies reviewing the use of nipple sparing mastectomy after reduction mammaplasty or mastopexy suggests that the NAC can survive even after having previously been circumferentially incised, suggesting revascularization across the periareolar scar.[56–58]

In many cases of repeated breast reduction, the NAC is in the ideal position and no pedicle is required so the risk of NAC necrosis is negligible. When the NAC needs to be transposed, a new pedicle can be used safely with minimal risk to the blood supply of the NAC, if designed carefully. The authors' method of pedicle selection limits the length-to-base width ratio of both the superior and superomedial dermoglandular flap to 1:1 (or less), providing a reliable blood supply to the NAC.

Skin Marking and Pedicle Selection

Markings are performed in the same manner as discussed previously for primary vertical scar reduction mammaplasty.[14,25] An important first step is to assess the position of the NAC (**Fig. 3**). If the NAC is in an adequate position relative to

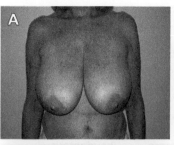
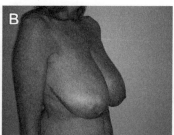
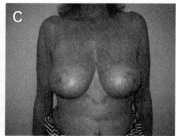
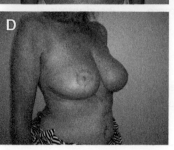

Fig. 1. (*A, B*) A 58-year-old woman who underwent previous bilateral breast reduction 34 years before repeated breast reduction had a lateral scar pattern, but the pedicles were unknown. (*C, D*) Result 8 months after vertical scar reduction mammaplasty with bilateral superomedial pedicles and vertically oriented, inferior wedge resections of breast tissue; 229 g were excised from the right breast, and 231 g were excised from the left breast. In addition, 120 mL were liposuctioned from the right breast and 140 mL from the left breast.

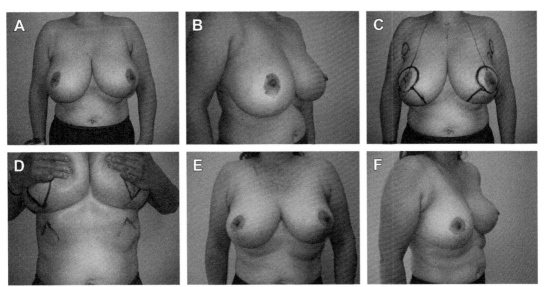

Fig. 2. (*A, B*) A 42-year-old woman who underwent her first bilateral breast reduction 22 years before and second breast reduction 17 years before having another repeated breast reduction. She had a vertical scar pattern, but the pedicles were unknown. (*C, D*) Bilateral superior pedicles are marked preoperatively. (*E, F*) Result 8 months after vertical scar reduction mammaplasty with bilateral superomedial pedicles and vertically oriented, inferior wedge resections of breast tissue; 571 g were excised from the right breast, and 528 g were excised from the left breast. In addition, 150 mL were liposuctioned from each breast.

the breast mound, a vertically oriented inferior wedge excision can be used without creation of a pedicle (**Fig. 4**). This is particularly useful in cases of pseudoptosis. In cases of the NAC requiring elevation, the authors use a partial thickness, superiorly based dermoglandular pedicle (**Fig. 5**). In the majority of repeated breast reduction cases, the NAC typically requires less than 5 cm of superior transposition. Up to this distance, the authors

believe it is safe to use a superior pedicle for cases in which the previous pedicle is unknown.[13] In cases that require greater transposition of the NAC, the authors have use a superomedial pedicle when the entire new NAC is below the blocking triangles.

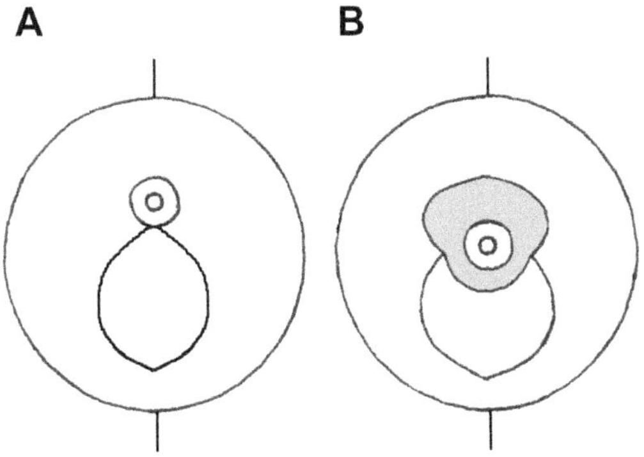

In repeated breast reduction cases correcting a size discrepancy between the two breasts, this asymmetry must be accounted for in the preoperative markings. The NAC on the larger side tends to sit higher postoperatively than was planned for preoperatively. Therefore, the NAC on the side requiring greater resection should be marked lower than the contralateral breast.[14] The authors believe this is due to the greater unweighting of the breast and greater recoil of the remaining breast tissue on the side that has a larger resection. In cases of repeated breast reduction with size asymmetry of greater than or equal to 100 g, the top of the planned new NAC on the larger side should be marked 1 cm to 2 cm lower than on the smaller side to account for differential unweighting of the breasts.

Fig. 3. Selection of the pedicle depends on the position of the NAC. (*A*) No pedicle is required with the ideal NAC position. (*B*) A superior pedicle is used with the low NAC position. (*From* Ahmad J, McIsaac SM, Lista F. Does knowledge of the initial technique affect outcomes after repeated breast reduction? Plast Reconstr Surg 2012;129(1):12; with permission.)

Infiltration

Infiltration of each breast with a wetting solution (1000 mL of Ringer lactate, 40 mL of 2% lidocaine, and 1 mL of 1:1000 epinephrine) helps minimize blood loss during dissection and liposuction. Infiltration is performed just deep to the skin along the

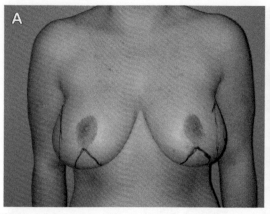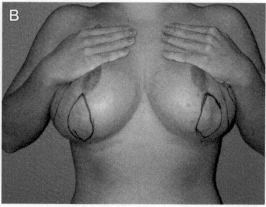

Fig. 4. (*A*) A 19-year-old woman, who underwent previous bilateral breast reduction 4 years before repeated breast reduction, had a medial J scar pattern, but the pedicles were unknown. The NACs are adequately positioned, so she was marked for bilateral vertically oriented, inferior wedge resections of breast tissue. (*B*) The inferior extent of skin resection is marked above the inframammary creases.

vertical limb incision lines as well as within the breast parenchyma. Minimal wetting solution should be infiltrated into the area of the planned dermoglandular pedicle. The lateral chest wall and preaxillary areas should also be infiltrated in preparation for liposuction.

De-epithelialization

During de-epithelialization of the dermoglandular pedicle, it is important to avoid damaging the blood vessels supporting the NAC, including the subdermal plexus. All efforts should be made to leave the deep dermis intact instead of removing the skin full thickness.

Excision of Breast Tissue

Excision of excess breast parenchyma using a vertically oriented inferior wedge resection allows for safe volume reduction while also creating a more narrow and projecting breast.[25,59]

If transposition of the NAC is required, a 2.5-cm to 3-cm thick superiorly based dermoglandular flap is created. It is important to ensure that this flap is left slightly thicker in repeated breast reduction cases to avoid injury to the vascular supply, which reliably runs approximately 1 cm deep to the dermis. When creating the medial parenchymal pillar, an incision should be made through the medial vertical limb straight down to just

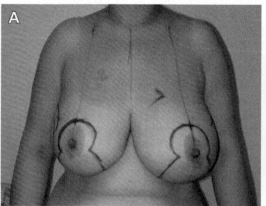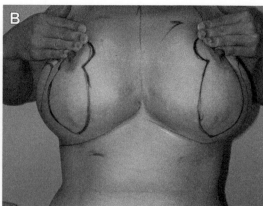

Fig. 5. (*A*) A 40-year-old woman who underwent previous bilateral breast reduction 5 years before repeated breast reduction had an inverted T scar pattern, but the pedicles were unknown. The NACs were located too low, so a mosque dome skin-marking pattern was drawn, and bilateral superior pedicles were used to transpose the bilateral NACs. (*B*) The inferior extent of the skin resection is marked above the inframammary creases. (*From* Ahmad J, McIsaac SM, Lista F. Does knowledge of the initial technique affect outcomes after repeated breast reduction? Plast Reconstr Surg 2012;129(1):14; with permission.)

superficial to the pectoralis fascia. Undermining of the medial pillar should be avoided to preserve medial fullness of the breast.

The majority of glandular excision in repeated breast reduction cases are from the central and lateral breast. Access to this tissue is created by developing a 2.5-cm thick lateral parenchymal pillar. Dissection can then be carried lateral and superolateral, with care to maintain a 2.5-cm thickness throughout, until the dissection reaches the lateral breast border–lateral chest wall transition point. After excision is complete, the superior and lateral skin flaps should feel smooth and even in thickness.

Finally, the tissue between the inferior edge of the vertical wound and the inframammary crease should be thinned under direct visualization to prevent dog ear formation. This also helps allow gathering of the skin of the vertical wound.

Liposuction

Liposuction is an important adjunct in cases of repeated breast reduction and is used in all cases.[5,9,13] Liposuction allows for volume reduction and contouring of the breast while minimizing the continuous undermining and preserving blood supply to the breast. Liposuction can be used on all areas of the breast based on the areas of excess determined preoperatively, although liposuction should be avoided in the area of the pedicle. Additionally, liposuction should be performed on the lateral fat compartment on the lateral chest wall to help define the lateral breast border. Liposuction is performed after parenchymal resection.

Closure

The inferior wedge resection of the redundant breast tissue that contributed to breast ptosis allows for the creation of medial and lateral parenchymal pillars. Suturing of these parenchymal pillars results in coning of the breast and is responsible for the pleasing projection associated with this technique. Wound closure is performed in 2 planes, including parenchymal pillar sutures and gathering of the skin of the vertical wound using 4-point boxing sutures. Usually, 2 parenchymal pillar sutures are used, but the inferior-most suture should be placed no closer than 4 cm from the inferior end of the incision. Placing the pillar sutures too close to the inferior end of the vertical wound opposes the gathering sutures and may lead to the formation a dog-ear at the inframammary crease. The 4-point boxing suture allows selective gathering of the vertical wound, leading to more control of the vertical

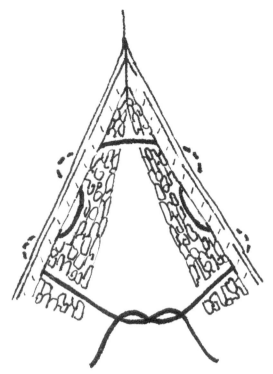

Fig. 6. A 4-point gathering box stitch is used to gather the skin of the vertical wound. (*From* Lista F, Ahmad J. Vertical scar reduction mammaplasty: 15-year experience including a review of 250 consecutive cases. Plast Reconstr Surg 2006;117(7):2157; with permission.)

scar (**Fig. 6**). Gathering of the skin assists in eliminating dog ears close to the inferior end of the vertical scar. Skin within 2 cm of the areola is not gathered to prevent distortion of the areola. After gathering of the skin, any gaping of the horizontal pleats caused by the 4-point boxing sutures along the vertical wound is corrected using inverted deep dermal sutures. Correction of these horizontal pleats is essential because they otherwise lead to small horizontal scars within the larger vertical scar. The vertical wound should be gathered enough to shorten the vertical scar such that it does not extend inferior to the inframammary crease.

SUMMARY

Recurrent or persistent macromastia after primary reduction mammaplasty can be a challenging problem. It is important to clearly define patients' concerns and goals as well as educate them on the limitations and risks of repeated breast reduction. Over the past 15 years, the authors have used a modified technique for vertical scar breast reduction in more than 40 patients and it has proved reliable and safe, even in cases where the original mammaplasty technique is unknown. For patients with pseudoptosis, a vertically oriented, inferior wedge resection can be safely excised, irrespective of the initial pedicle. For patients with ptosis in whom the NAC needs to be transposed superiorly, a carefully planned and de-epithelialized superior pedicle should be used. This pedicle combined with a vertically oriented, inferior wedge resection, limiting the amount of undermining of breast tissue, helps maintain blood supply to the remaining breast tissue. Additionally, liposuction is an important adjunct to achieve volume reduction while limiting the amount of dissection during repeated breast reduction.

REFERENCES

1. American Society for Aesthetic Plastic Surgery. Cosmetic surgery national data bank statistics. 2014. Available at: http://www.surgery.org/sites/default/files/2014-Stats.pdf. Accessed May 25, 2015.
2. Herman S, Hoffman S, Kahn S. Revisional surgery after reduction mammaplasty. Plast Reconstr Surg 1975;55(4):422–7.
3. Hoffman S. Recurrent deformities following reduction mammaplasty and correction of breast asymmetry. Plast Reconstr Surg 1986;78(1):55–62.
4. Pandeya NK. Inferior pedicle technique for reduction mammaplasty after a strombeck reduction. Plast Reconstr Surg 1996;97(6):1306.
5. Lejour M. Vertical mammaplasty as secondary surgery after other techniques. Aesthetic Plast Surg 1997;21(6):403–7.
6. Hudson DA, Skoll PJ. Repeat reduction mammaplasty. Plast Reconstr Surg 1999;104(2):401–8.
7. Losee JE, Caldwell EH, Serletti JM. Secondary reduction mammaplasty: is using a different pedicle safe? Plast Reconstr Surg 2000;106(5):1004–8.
8. Patel SP, Brown DL, Cederna PS. Repeated bilateral reduction mammaplasty: a 12-year experience. Plast Reconstr Surg 2010;126(5):263e–4e.
9. Sultan MR, Schwartz JA, Smith ML, et al. Revision of wise pattern breast reductions with vertical procedures. Ann Plast Surg 2013;71(3):300–3.
10. Skoll PJ, Hudson DA. The safety of a different pedicle in secondary reduction mammaplasty. Plast Reconstr Surg 2001;108(4):1086.
11. Spear SL. Secondary reduction mammaplasty: is using a different pedicle safe? by Joseph E. Losee, M.D., Elethea H. Caldwell, M.D., and Joseph M. Serletti, M.D. Plast Reconstr Surg 2000;106(5):1009–10.
12. Rohrich RJ, Thornton JF, Sorokin ES. Recurrent mammary hyperplasia: current concepts. Plast Reconstr Surg 2003;111(1):387–93.
13. Ahmad J, McIsaac SM, Lista F. Does knowledge of the initial technique affect outcomes after repeated breast reduction? Plast Reconstr Surg 2012;129(1):11–8.
14. Lista F, Austin RE, Singh Y, et al. Vertical scar reduction mammaplasty. Plast Reconstr Surg 2015;136(1):23–5.
15. Regnault P, Daniel RK. Breast reduction. In: Regnault P, Daniel RK, editors. Aesthetic plastic surgery principles and techniques. Boston (MA): Little, Brown and Co; 1984. p. 499–538.
16. Kocak E, Carruthers KH, McMahan JD. A reliable method for the preoperative estimation of tissue to be removed during reduction mammaplasty. Plast Reconstr Surg 2011;127(3):1059–64.
17. Appel JZ 3rd, Wendel JJ, Zellner EG, et al. Association between preoperative measurements and resection weight in patients undergoing reduction mammaplasty. Ann Plast Surg 2010;64(5):512–5.
18. Descamps MJL, Landau AG, Lazarus D, et al. A formula determining resection weights for reduction mammaplasty. Plast Reconstr Surg 2008;121(2):397–400.
19. Eder M, Grabhorn A, Waldenfels FV, et al. Prediction of breast resection weight in reduction mammaplasty based on 3-dimensional surface imaging. Surg Innov 2013;20(4):356–64.
20. Pechter EA. A new method for determining bra size and predicting postaugmentation breast size. Plast Reconstr Surg 1998;102(4):1259–65.
21. Regnault P. Breast ptosis. Definition and treatment. Clin Plast Surg 1976;3(2):193–203.
22. Brown RH, Izaddoost S, Bullocks JM. Preventing the "bottoming out" and 'star-gazing' phenomena in inferior pedicle breast reduction with an acellular dermal matrix internal brassiere. Aesthetic Plast Surg 2010;34(6):760–7.
23. Mizgala CL, MacKenzie KM. Breast reduction outcome study. Ann Plast Surg 2000;44(2):125–33.
24. Bouwer LR, van der Biezen JJ, Spronk CA, et al. Vertical scar versus the inverted-T scar reduction mammaplasty: a 10-year follow-up. J Plast Reconstr Aesthet Surg 2012;65(10):1298–304.
25. Lista F, Ahmad J. Vertical scar reduction mammaplasty: a 15-year experience including a review of 250 consecutive cases. Plast Reconstr Surg 2006;117(7):2152–65.
26. Choi M, Unger J, Small K, et al. Defining the kinetics of breast pseudoptosis after reduction mammaplasty. Ann Plast Surg 2009;62(5):518–22.
27. Small KH, Tepper OM, Unger JG, et al. Re-defining pseudoptosis from a 3D perspective after short scar-medial pedicle reduction mammaplasty. J Plast Reconstr Aesthet Surg 2010;63(2):346–53.
28. Quan M, Fadl A, Small K, et al. Defining pseudoptosis (bottoming out) 3 years after short-scar medial pedicle breast reduction. Aesthetic Plast Surg 2011;35(3):357–64.

29. Oni G, Saint-Cyr M, Maia M, et al. Dermolipectomy of the lateral thoracic fat compartment in secondary breast reconstruction revision: anatomical and clinical results. J Plast Reconstr Aesthet Surg 2012; 65(2):201–6.

30. Kerrigan CL, Collins ED, Kim HM, et al. Reduction mammaplasty: defining medical necessity. Med Decis Making 2002;22(3):208–17.

31. Spector JA, Kleinerman R, Culliford AT 4th, et al. The vertical reduction mammaplasty: a prospective analysis of patient outcomes. Plast Reconstr Surg 2006; 117(2):374–81.

32. Kerrigan CL, Collins ED, Striplin D, et al. The health burden of breast hypertrophy. Plast Reconstr Surg 2001;108(6):1591–9.

33. Ekman I, Swedberg K, Taft C, et al. Person-centered care – ready for prime time. Eur J Cardiovasc Nurs 2011;10(4):248–51.

34. Cruz-Korchin N, Korchin L. Breast-feeding after vertical mammaplasty with medial pedicle. Plast Reconstr Surg 2004;114(4):890–4.

35. Chang DS, McGrath MH. Management of benign tumors of the adolescent breast. Plast Reconstr Surg 2007;120(1):13e–9e.

36. Hoppe IC, Patel PP, Singer-Granick CJ, et al. Virginal mammary hypertrophy: a meta-analysis and treatment algorithm. Plast Reconstr Surg 2011;127(6): 2224–31.

37. Neinstein LS. Breast disease in adolescents and young women. Pediatr Clin North Am 1999;46(3): 607–29.

38. Pruthi S, Jones K. Nonsurgical management of fibroadenoma and virginal breast hypertrophy. Semin Plast Surg 2013;27(1):62–6.

39. Brown MH, Weinberg M, Chong N, et al. A cohort study of breast cancer risk in breast reduction patients. Plast Reconstr Surg 1999;103(6):1674–81.

40. Boice JD, Persson I, Brinton LA, et al. Breast cancer following breast reduction surgery in Sweden. Plast Reconstr Surg 2000;106(4):755–62.

41. Boice JD, Friis S, McLaughlin JK, et al. Cancer following breast reduction surgery in Denmark. Cancer Causes Control 1997;8(2):253–8.

42. Baasch M, Nielsen SF, Engholm G, et al. Breast cancer incidence subsequent to surgical reduction of the female breast. Br J Cancer 1996;73(7):961–3.

43. Manahan MA, Buretta KJ, Chang D, et al. An outcomes analysis of 2142 breast reduction procedures. Ann Plast Surg 2015;74(3):289–92.

44. Srinivasaiah N, Iwuchukwu OC, Stanley PRW, et al. Risk factors for complications following breast reduction: results from a randomized control trial. Breast J 2014;20(3):274–8.

45. Robert G, Duhamel A, Alet JM, et al. Complications of breast reduction about 715 breasts. Ann Chir Plast Esthet 2014;59(2):97–102.

46. Lewin R, Göransson M, Elander A, et al. Risk factors for complications after breast reduction surgery. J Plast Surg Hand Surg 2014;48(1):10–4.

47. Bikhchandani J, Varma SK, Henderson HP. Is it justified to refuse breast reduction to smokers? J Plast Reconstr Aesthet Surg 2007;60(9):1050–4.

48. Pluvy I, Garrido I, Pauchot J, et al. Smoking and plastic surgery, part I. pathophysiological aspects: update and proposed recommendations. Ann Chir Plast Esthet 2015;60(1):e3–13.

49. Rinker B. The evils of nicotine: an evidence-based guide to smoking and plastic surgery. Ann Plast Surg 2013;70(5):599–605.

50. Eder M, Klöppel M, Müller D, et al. 3-D analysis of breast morphology changes after inverted t-scar and vertical-scar reduction mammaplasty over 12 months. J Plast Reconstr Aesthet Surg 2013;66(6): 776–86.

51. van Deventer PV. The blood supply to the nipple-areola complex of the human mammary gland. Aesthetic Plast Surg 2004;28(6):393–8.

52. van Deventer PV, Page BJ, Graewe FR. The safety of pedicles in breast reduction and mastopexy procedures. Aesthetic Plast Surg 2008;32(2):307–12.

53. Seitz IA, Nixon AT, Friedewald SM, et al. "NAC-somes": a new classification system of the blood supply to the nipple areola complex (NAC) based on diagnostic breast MRI exams. J Plast Reconstr Aesthet Surg 2015;68(6):792–9.

54. le Roux CM, Pan WR, Matousek SA, et al. Preventing venous congestion of the nipple-areola complex: an anatomical guide to preserving essential venous drainage networks. Plast Reconstr Surg 2011; 127(3):1073–9.

55. Michelle le Roux C, Kiil BJ, Pan WR, et al. Preserving the neurovascular supply in the hall-findlay superomedial pedicle breast reduction: an anatomical study. J Plast Reconstr Aesthet Surg 2010;63(4):655–62.

56. Alperovich M, Tanna N, Blechman KM, et al. Nipple-sparing mastectomy in patients with a history of reduction mammaplasty or mastopexy. Plast Reconstr Surg 2013;131(5):962–7.

57. Spear SL, Rothman SJ, Seiboth LA, et al. Breast reconstruction using a staged nipple-sparing mastectomy following mastopexy or reduction. Plast Reconstr Surg 2012;129(3):572–81.

58. Frederick MJ, Lin AM, Neuman R, et al. Nipple-sparing mastectomy in patients with previous breast surgery: comparative analysis of 775 immediate breast reconstructions. Plast Reconstr Surg 2015;135(6):954e–62e.

59. Ahmad J, Lista F. Vertical scar reduction mammaplasty: the fate of nipple-areola complex position and inferior pole length. Plast Reconstr Surg 2008; 121(4):1084–91.

Management of the High-Riding Nipple After Breast Reduction

Scott L. Spear, MD[a],*, Frank P. Albino, MD[b]

KEYWORDS

• Management • High-riding nipple • Breast reduction

KEY POINTS

- Preventing excessive nipple elevation following reduction mammaplasty is far easier and more successful than correcting the problem.
- The key to avoiding overelevation of the nipple is to allow sufficient skin from the upper breast border to the top of the planned new areola window, a minimum of 8 cm and frequently 10 cm in larger breasts.
- Favor the superior, medial, or superomedial pedicles with vertical closure of glandular flaps to improve breast coning and projection, which likely reduces the risk of the reduced breast bottoming out. When bottoming out has occurred, correction can include a lower pole reduction including a transverse excision as a crescent or inverted T but avoiding further elevation of the nipple.
- In patients with apparent nipple malposition accentuated by upper pole deficiency, an augmentation with an implant or fat grafting can improve superior pole projection and indirectly lower or seem to lower the nipple-areolar position on the breast.
- In those patients whereby the nipple to sternal notch or nipple to upper breast border has been seriously shortened, it may be necessary to directly move the nipple-areolar complex by transposition, V-Y inferior advancement, or reciprocal skin grafting in addition to other steps, such as upper pole volume enhancement.

INTRODUCTION

The high-riding nipple-areolar complex (NAC) is a potential complication of cosmetic or reconstructive breast procedures. In its milder forms, it is very common and results in an upward-facing nipple sitting above the breast equator and above the point of maximal projection. This milder form often goes unnoticed. In its more severe presentations, it can be very disfiguring and embarrassing.

Breast reduction and mastopexy, in particular, are routinely designed to elevate the NAC but often may result in an NAC that appears elevated more than ideal or anticipated in the preoperative plan. The site for proper nipple position during a reduction mammaplasty should be carefully selected in order to ensure the NAC ultimately is positioned at or near the most projected area of the breast, regardless of the dermo-glandular pedicle chosen or skin pattern selected. With a real potential for NAC displacement, some surgeons endorse marking the new nipple position 1.5 to 1.75 cm below the most projected area of the breast intraoperatively.[1] Ahmad and Lista[2] followed 46 consecutive women following vertical

No funding was used in the preparation of this article. Dr S.L. Spear is a paid consultant to Lifecell Corporation and to Allergan Corporation. Dr F.P. Albino does not have any affiliations to declare.
[a] Private Practice, Washington, DC, USA; [b] Department of Plastic Surgery, MedStar Georgetown University Hospital, 3800 Reservoir Road, Northwest, Washington, DC 20007, USA
* Corresponding author. 5454 Wisconsin Avenue, Suite #1210, Chevy Chase, MD 20815.
E-mail address: scottspear@drscottspear.com

Clin Plastic Surg 43 (2016) 395–401
http://dx.doi.org/10.1016/j.cps.2015.12.008
0094-1298/16/$ – see front matter © 2016 Elsevier Inc. All rights reserved.

plasticsurgery.theclinics.com

scar reduction mammaplasty and found that the nipple-areola complex 4 years after surgery was located on average 1 cm higher compared with the planned position by preoperative skin markings. Similarly, Keck and colleagues[3] note that a planned notch-to-nipple distance of 22 to 24 cm resulted in an immediate postoperative notch-to-nipple distance of 18 to 20 cm (P value .01). Furthermore, over the next 3 months, the nipple-to-notch distance continued to change by an additional 17%.

The importance of achieving a suitable NAC position following reduction mammaplasty develops from the real potential for a high-riding outcome and the difficulty in addressing this complication. The challenge in developing an operative plan to adequately address the high-riding NAC to the satisfaction of the surgeon and patients is based on the nature and degree of displacement and cannot be overstated. Part of this difficulty stems from the desire to avoid leaving scars that lie above the superior edge of the NAC and the limited amount of skin available between the nipple and the clavicle. Several strategies have been described to address these issues, including elevating the inframammary fold (IMF) and the breast parenchyma, expanding the skin superior to the NAC, and directly repositioning the nipple by excising it and grafting it in a more appropriate location.[4–7] The high-riding nipple presents a complicated reconstructive challenge. Appreciating its cause and the available corrective surgical options may help surgeons, on the one hand, minimize the likelihood of creating malpositioned nipples and may, on the other hand, help select an appropriate intervention to correct the problem when it occurs.

SUMMARY/DISCUSSION

Nipple position and the overall appearance of the breast can be quite variable among those deemed high. Evaluating the breast aesthetically does not necessarily necessitate more than a basic appreciation for the overall breast shape and proportion. Nipple position and symmetry are critical elements to consider in the evaluation of breast appearance before or following surgery. **Fig. 1** demonstrates bilateral high-riding NACs for this 58-year-old patient, 6 years following Wise pattern reduction mammaplasty using an inferior pedicle. Unhappy with the current positioning of her nipples, she presented to the authors' office seeking revision. Note the short distance from the superior border of the breast to the top of the areola leading to a displeasing overall breast contour and a nipple malpositioned to the extent that it might become exposed inadvertently.

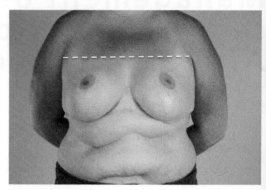

Fig. 1. A 58-year-old woman presents 6 years following reduction mammaplasty seeking improvement in her current nipple position. Note the short distance from the superior boarder of the breast to the top of the areola leading to a displeasing overall NAC position (*white dotted line* defines the approximate upper border of the breast silhouette).

Clearly a difficult problem to address, it is best to avoid the creation of a high-riding nipple following reduction mammaplasty all together. The most important lesson for treatment of the superiorly displaced NAC following reduction mammaplasty is that prevention is far easier than the solution. Toward this goal, it is critical to sufficiently evaluate the preoperative breast when selecting and subsequently marking the new nipple position (**Figs. 2** and **3**). Moving the nipple cranially is often a desired effect of a breast reduction; however, selecting a new target position requires sophisticated planning. Transposition of the IMF continues to prove to be the most widely accepted approach for selecting new nipple position; however, this approach may be fraught with problems in the setting of a pendulant and ptotic breast, gigantomastia, or when the breast footprint begins low on the torso. Rather the IMF transposition at the level of the breast meridian should be used as a guide to mark the new nipple position. The authors think it is equally or more important to ensure there is sufficient skin from the upper breast border to the top of the planned new areola window, a minimum of 8 cm and frequently 10 cm in larger breasts. Increasing the breast projection will also aid in ensuring the nipple position does not further move cranially. A superior, medial or superomedial pedicle is preferred in order to allow for resection of inferior parenchyma, minimizing the risk of bottoming out, and allowing for closure of medial and lateral glandular flaps to improve breast coning and projection. These pedicles promote superior pole fullness and, thereby, safeguard against the development of a high-riding nipple.

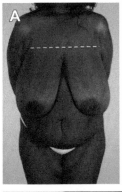
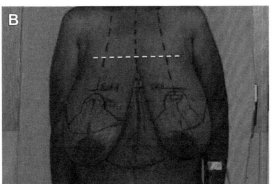
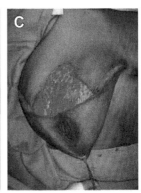
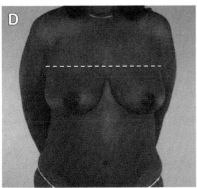

Fig. 2. (*A*, *B*) A 36-year-old woman presents with macromastia seeking reduction mammaplasty. A Wise pattern is marked (*B*) with the new nipple position planned 2 cm below the transposed IMF at a point 10 cm from the upper breast border as shown by the dotted white line. A superomedial pedicle is marked in green, but ultimately the reduction was performed with a free-nipple graft. (*C*, *D*) The recipient site for the nipple graft is maintained on a broad thick superior de-epithelized dermoglandular pedicle (*C*). Following removal of nearly 2000 g from each breast, the subsequent medial and lateral glandular pillars are loosely imbricated and reapproximated for additional projection and support. At the 6-month follow-up, the overall breast size and shape is much improved with appropriate if not ideal nipple position with maintenance of an appropriate distance from the nipple to the upper breast border.

If the nipple is elevated too high and patients are dissatisfied, there are a few approaches that may be undertaken. Scar location, absolute nipple position (sternal notch-to-nipple distance or nipple-to-IMF distance), IMF position, location of breast volume, blood supply, breast skin elasticity/quantity, and previous radiation therapy are all considerations in selecting the most

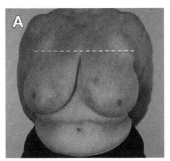
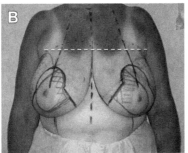
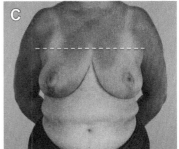
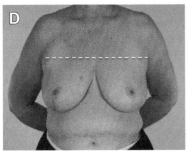

Fig. 3. (*A*, *B*) A 51-year-old woman presents with macromastia seeking reduction mammaplasty. A Wise pattern is marked (*B*) with the new nipple position planned at the transposed IMF at a point 8 cm from the upper breast border as shown by the dotted white line. A superomedial pedicle is marked in red. (*C*, *D*) Two-month (*C*) and 1-year (*D*) follow-up following reduction mammaplasty demonstrating nipple position with maintenance of an appropriate distance from the nipple to the upper breast border.

appropriate surgical approach. Based on these factors, excising and discarding the nipple may rarely in extreme cases be the best option, such as prior radiation therapy, unfavorable scars, or a very tight skin envelope. Excision can be followed by nipple reconstruction at the same time or at a later date in a staged fashion. On the other hand, in more encouraging situations, various techniques to reposition the native nipple may be pursued.

There are few options available to correct the NAC when the nipple is positioned too superiorly. The authors have found that an important step in selecting a surgical solution is to make a diagnosis, look at the nipple position relative to the entire breast shape, attempt to visualize the alternative approaches, and ultimately select the best solution. Would patients benefit more from addressing the position of the breast mound, both the nipple and the breast mound, or just the nipple in isolation?

INDIRECT CORRECTION OF THE NIPPLE-AREOLA COMPLEX POSITION

Indirect approaches to nipple position addressing only the breast mound may be the preferred solution in the setting of a normal or near-normal nipple-to-sternal notch distance, a long nipple-to-IMF distance (≥8 cm), a bottomed-out breast or implant with the device sitting below the IMF scar, or a depleted upper pole. For these cases of a relative high-riding nipple, the IMF can be raised or the upper breast pole may be expanded to give the appearance of lowering the NAC.

INFERIOR BREAST PARENCHYMA RESECTION

A wedge resection of inferior breast parenchyma allows for shortening of the nipple-to-IMF distance and may prevent bottoming out of breast parenchyma. In decreasing the amount of glandular tissue below the nipple, it effectively improves the overall nipple position by or shortening the breast around it. **Fig. 4** demonstrates the successful implementation of inferior breast parenchyma resection as a small-volume breast reduction in the setting of bilateral, high NACs notable for long nipple-to-fold distances greater than 10 cm.

SUPERIOR BREAST VOLUME ADDITION

Upper pole expansion may be achieved through insertion of an implant or lipoaugmentation. If the skin envelope will not accommodate additional upper pole volume, tissue expansion may be required before the definitive implant. Colwell and colleagues[6] have described the option of infraclavicular tissue expansion in 3 patients found to have high-riding NACs following reduction mammaplasty or augmentation/mastopexy. This technique modestly increases the sternal notch-to-nipple distance but does not require direct movement of the NAC. **Figs. 5** and **6** demonstrate improvement to breast shape and nipple position following dual-plane breast augmentation in the setting of a deficient upper breast pole and high-riding nipple after reduction mammaplasty. This result may require lower pole support using an acellular dermal matrix (see **Fig. 6**) as necessitated by the current lower

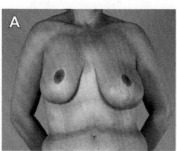
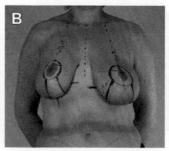
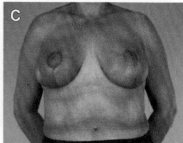
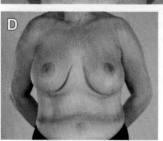

Fig. 4. (A) A 49-year-old woman presents 3 years following Wise pattern, inferior pedicle breast reduction concerned with bottoming out and overly elevated NACs, the right higher than the left. (B) The plan for correction included an asymmetric inferior dermoglandular resection executed as circumvertical reductions without further elevation of the nipple. Right and left resection weights were 200 g and 300 g, respectively. Two-month (C) and (D) 1-year postoperative follow-up photographs demonstrate marked improvements in breast symmetry, size, shape, and nipple position. Although the nipple position is much improved, it is still higher than ideal.

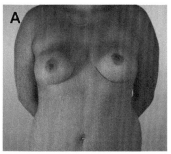
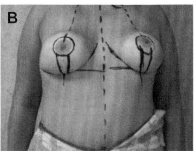
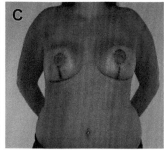
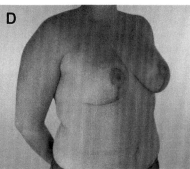

Fig. 5. (*A, B*) A 23-year-old woman with history of a tubular breast deformity who underwent a right mastopexy and left small-volume breast reduction presents now with a mildly superiorly displaced left NAC and bilaterally deficient upper breast poles (*A*). Preoperative markings for single-stage augmentation and revision mastopexy (*B*). (*C, D*) Early postoperative result (*C*) following dual-plane augmentation with Allergan Style 68MP saline 270-mL (Allergan pic, Dublin, Ireland) implants followed by mastopexy. Six-month follow-up (*D*) demonstrates improved nipple position and upper breast contour.

pole soft tissue and planned parenchymal reshaping.

DIRECT CORRECTION OF THE NIPPLE-AREOLA COMPLEX POSITION

Alternatively, direct nipple movement through a skin graft or reciprocal transposition flap is preferred in the setting of a short sternal notch-to-nipple distance combined with a reasonable nipple-to-IMF distance (5–7 cm). Classified as absolute malposition, the nipple can be moved directly by excision of adjacent skin, grafting to a more favorable location, or transposition as a flap.[6–10] When nipple malposition is caused by elements of both relative and absolute nipple displacement, the operative intervention can correct these elements either simultaneously or

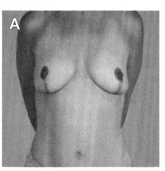
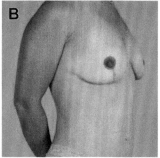
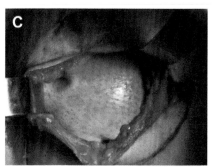
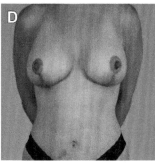

Fig. 6. A 34-year-old woman presents 2 years following breast reduction and 35-lb weight loss now with deflated breasts seeking improvement to her nipple position and breast shape (*A, B*). She underwent a staged reconstruction. First, a dual-plane breast augmentation was performed using McGhan Style 15 286-mL silicone implants and AlloDerm reinforcement over the lower breast pole (*C, D*).

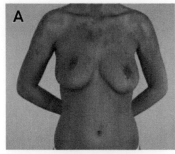
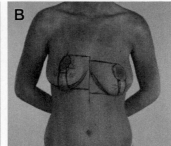
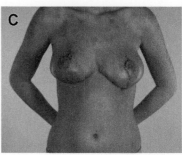
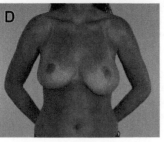

Fig. 7. A 24-year-old woman presents 6 years following reduction mammaplasty with unsatisfactory breast shape and nipple malposition worse on the right side (*A*). A Wise pattern, small-volume reduction is planned to remove some inferior breast tissue along with a right breast V-Y inferior advancement to move the NAC downward (*B*). Early postoperative result (*C*) and 1-year follow-up (*D*) demonstrate improvement in nipple position, acceptable scar placement, and better overall breast shape, although the left breast has recurrent glandular ptosis, which should be correctable.

separately in a staged fashion. Whether to initially address the breast or the nipple should be dictated by the more severe or more easily correctable deformity. Generally, it is preferable to correct the position of the breast mound first.

V-Y INFERIOR NIPPLE REPOSITIONING

Using local tissue rearrangement, direct nipple repositioning may also be achieved with a V-Y advancement using a flap to advance the NAC distally. This technique does place incisions over the superior breast pole; however, it can be successful in achieving improved NAC position for patients with an acceptable, or even shortened, nipple-to-fold distance. **Fig. 7** illustrates the use of a unilateral V-Y inferior nipple repositioning in

combination with a small-volume, lower pole breast reduction to elevate the IMF, reshape the breast parenchyma, and provide greater upper pole fullness.

RECIPROCAL TRANSPOSITION FLAPS

Three technical points need to be emphasized in the performance of the reciprocal transposition flap. First, flap elevation is performed in the deep subcutaneous plane, just superficial to the capsule. Manipulation should be sharp and minimally traumatic. Second, the flaps should be rotated and inset with as little tension as possible. Consequently, trimming of standing cones (dog ears) should be avoided or minimized to preserve flap perfusion. Third, this procedure should be approached with caution in irradiated patients. Any suggestion of flap ischemia in the postoperative

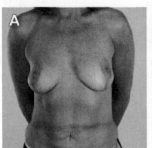
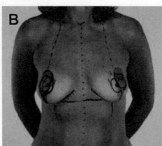
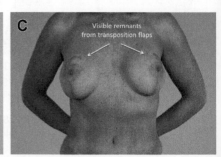

Fig. 8. A 49-year-old woman presents with widened, superiorly displaced NACs and upper pole deflation 4 years following small-volume reduction mammaplasty (*A*). In order to correct the nipple malpositions, each nipple is marked for repositioning using reciprocal transposition flaps (*B*). An augmentation is performed at the same time to address the breast deflation. (*C*) One year following bilateral nipple repositioning with reciprocal transposition flaps combined with bilateral dual-plane breast augmentation.

period may benefit from hyperbaric oxygen therapy to improve flap perfusion. **Fig. 8** demonstrates the results of bilateral reciprocal transposition flaps in the setting of bilateral augmentation mastopexy for nipple malposition following breast reduction.

REFERENCES

1. Altuntas ZK, Kamburoglu HO, Yavuz N, et al. Long-term changes in nipple-areolar complex position and inferior pole length in superomedial pedicle inverted 't' scar reduction mammoplasty. Aesthetic Plast Surg 2015;39(3):325–30.

2. Ahmad J, Lista F. Vertical scar reduction mammaplasty: the fate of nipple-areola complex position and inferior pole length. Plast Reconstr Surg 2008; 121:1084–91.

3. Keck M, Kayne K, Thieme I, et al. Vertical mammoplasty: postoperative changes, complications, and patient evaluation. Can J Plast Surg 2007; 15(1):41–3.

4. Millard DR Jr, Mullin WR, Lesavoy MA. Secondary correction of the too-high areola and nipple after mammaplasty. Plast Reconstr Surg 1976;58: 568–72.

5. Elsahy NI. Correction of abnormally high nipples after reduction mammaplasty. Aesthetic Plast Surg 1990;14:21–6.

6. Colwell AS, May JW Jr, Slavin SA. Lowering the postoperative high-riding nipple. Plast Reconstr Surg 2007;120:596–9.

7. Spear SL, Hoffman S. Relocation of the displaced nipple-areola by reciprocal skin grafts. Plast Reconstr Surg 1998;101:1355–8.

8. Frenkiel BA, Pacifico MD, Ritz M, et al. A solution to the high-riding nipple-areola complex. Aesthetic Plast Surg 2010;34(4):525–7.

9. Mohmand H, Naasan A. Double U-plasty for correction of geometric malposition of the nipple-areola complex. Plast Reconstr Surg 2002;109(6): 2019–22.

10. van Straalen WR, van Trier AJ, Groenvelt F. Correction of the post-burn malpositioned nipple-areola complex by transposition of two subcutaneous pedicled flaps. Br J Plast Surg 2000;53(5): 406–9.

Management of the Ischemic Nipple–Areola Complex After Breast Reduction

Alberto Rancati, MD, PhD*, Marcelo Irigo, MD, PhD,
Claudio Angrigiani, MD

KEYWORDS

• Areolar • Nipple • Necrosis • Ischemia • Management

KEY POINTS

• The anatomy of breast circulation as a key element to prevent nipple–areolar complex (NAC) ischemia and necrosis.
• Ischemia detection during the operative procedure to enable reperfusion maneuvers is important.
• Reperfusion techniques are described as essential to revert NAC sufferance.
• NAC grafting as last option in salvage attempt, and as primary indication.
• NAC reconstruction with different techniques and with synthetic materials is described.

 Video content accompanies this article at www.plastic.theclinics.com

INTRODUCTION

Partial or total nipple necrosis after breast reduction surgery can be a devastating complication for the patient and the surgeon (**Figs. 1** and **2**). Frequent monitoring of the nipple–areola complex (NAC) and early identification of vascular compromise followed by appropriate action may prevent total NAC loss. Intraoperative pale appearance of the NAC complex can be the initial sign indicating that "something is wrong."[1–3]

Different maneuvers other than tissue resection that are performed during breast reduction surgery can alter NAC vitality and lead to ischemia and partial/total loss, areolar sufferance, nipple projection loss, and/or hypopigmentation.[4–6] This situation can arise independent of the technique.[7–9]

NAC necrosis has been reported in 2% of breast reduction cases and in 1% of mastopexy cases; epidermolysis with blisterlike formation owing to intradermal or subdermal edema may result in 5% to 11% of cases.[1,10]

ANATOMIC CONSIDERATIONS

An important element for understanding the possibility of NAC ischemia and necrosis is awareness of breast and NAC vascular anatomy.[11,12] Any surgical maneuver involving the breast parenchyma will alter not only its architecture but its blood supply as well. Detaching the parenchyma from the pectoralis fascia is not necessary during reduction procedures; this alters not only the vascularization but also the breast innervation, leading to unnecessary complications.[13,14] Regardless of the

The authors declare no conflict of interest. This article is for educational purposes only, and the artwork used is original.
Department of Oncoplastic Surgery, Instituto Oncologico Henry Moore, University of Buenos Aires, Argentina
* Corresponding author. 19333 Collins Avenue #2302, Ocean One Building, Sunny Isles Beach, FL 33160.
E-mail address: rancati@gmail.com

Clin Plastic Surg 43 (2016) 403–414
http://dx.doi.org/10.1016/j.cps.2015.12.011
0094-1298/16/$ – see front matter

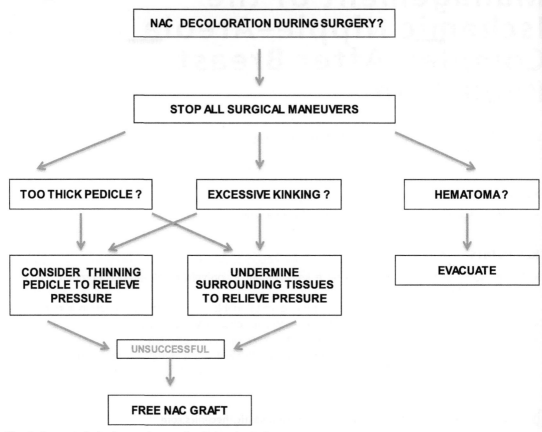

Fig. 1. Suspected nipple–areola complex ischemia during surgery.

chosen pedicle, the reduction technique, and resected breast parenchyma, the remaining breast tissue and NAC can be mobilized to the final position without detachment from the pectoralis fascia (Video 1). This can be done with inverted pyramidal resections, thereby avoiding the remaining dead spaces.[15,16]

Vascular Nutrition of the Breast

- Internal and external mammary systems (**Fig. 3**);
- Thoracoacromial artery with corresponding perforators;
- Intercostal perforator vessels;
- Lateral thoracic system; and
- Supraclavicular branches.

Another key element to keep in mind during breast reduction revisions is the patient history related to previous breast surgeries and access to surgical protocols (it is ideal if pictures are available). It is impossible to determine the surgical strategies previously used based only on the visible skin scar pattern alone; information on the surgery performed over the parenchyma

related to the original breast size, resected tissue volume, selected NAC pedicle, original existing relations of the NAC, and surgery dates is fundamental to prevent NAC loss during a revision surgery (**Fig. 4**).[16–19]

RISK FACTORS CONTRIBUTING TO NIPPLE–AREOLA COMPLEX NECROSIS

NAC ischemia and necrosis occurs more frequently in cases involving large reductions (resection >1000 g), where a long pedicle is created to carry NAC perfusion, and folding during closure can stress the circulation.[12,20–22]

Be Alert to

- Length of pedicle (>10 cm mobilization);
- Large reductions (>1000 g);
- Excessive pedicle folding, kinking, or malrotation;
- Excessive thinning of the pedicle;
- Dense gland pedicle (compression);
- Simultaneous augmentation, mastopexy, and reduction with implant compression; and

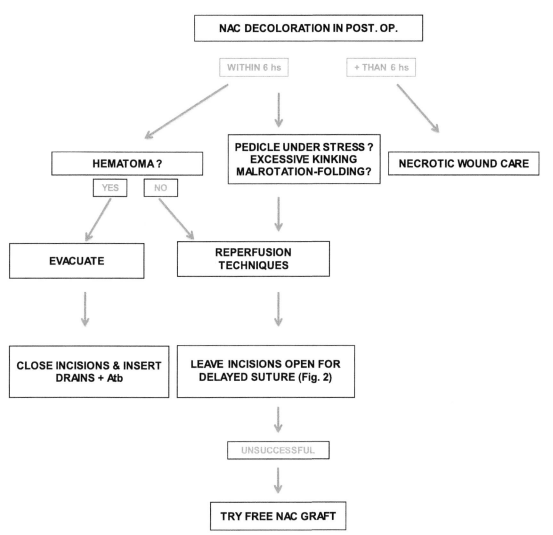

Fig. 2. Detected nipple–areola complex ischemia after surgery.

- Reoperative reduction or mastopexy with an unknown initial pedicle.
- Malignancies or immunomodulating medication.

ASSOCIATED RISK FACTORS

The following are individual conditions that can increase the risk of NAC necrosis:

- Body mass index >30 kg/m^2;
- Diabetes;
- Past history of poor wound healing;
- Heavy smoking;
- Simultaneous augmentation and mastopexy;
- Previous radiotherapy-chemotherapy;
- Steroid use;
- Previous scars around the NAC;
- Post–bariatric surgery malnutrition;
- Genetic predisposition to thrombosis; and

PREOPERATIVE CONTROL

We believe that sometimes an augmented risk can be present associated with the patient's personal history. To diminish the possibilities of NAC ischemia and necrosis, we suggest that the following items must be checked before surgery and be registered in every preoperative reduction mammaplasty patient.[23,24]

- Nutritional state and serum albumin level;
- Hemogram;
- Recent weight loss or gain; and
- Pulmonary function.

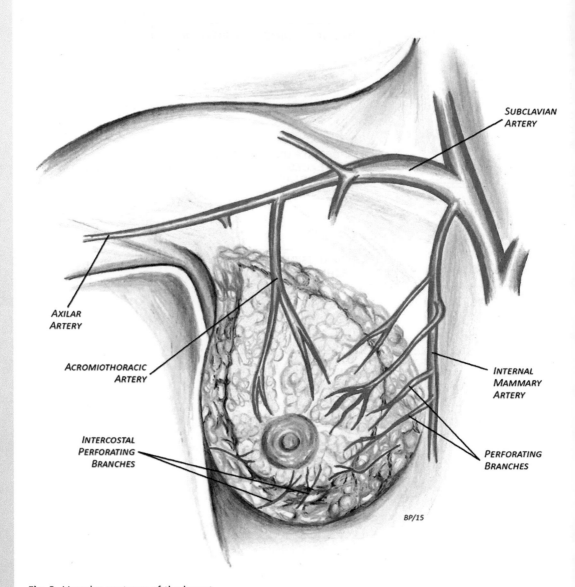

Fig. 3. Vascular anatomy of the breast.

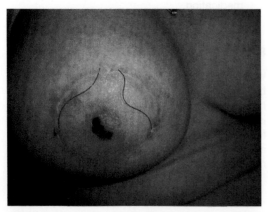

Fig. 4. Partial nipple necrosis after periareolar revision after 6 months of inverted T, mastopexy.

INTRAOPERATIVE EVALUATION
Vitality of the Nipple–Areola Complex During Closure Is an Important Factor to Be Checked in Every Mammaplasty Procedure

Vitality of the NAC can be preserved with appropriate care of the mentioned anatomic concepts during surgery; however, even with care taken regarding pedicle selection and a perfect technique, NAC vitality must be rechecked after surgical closure to avoid this complication. At this last moment, NAC vitality evolution is decided.[25,26]

Excessive pedicle folding, compression, areolar tightening, or a bulky pedicle can stress the circulation; therefore, if NAC ischemia is suspected, incisions must be opened, sutures released, and the pedicle examined. In some cases, the pedicle must be reduced in volume, and the circulation must be reevaluated.[3,27] If these maneuvers improve NAC perfusion, wound reclosure must be attempted, and the vitality reevaluated. If the circulation remains deficient, the pedicle might be trimmed further, and in some cases, the incisions may be left open (**Fig. 5**).

Sometimes, alteration in NAC color may provide an indication regarding the problem and the required rescue maneuvers.[4,28]

- Complete arterial insufficiency? White color.
- Incomplete arterial insufficiency? Grayish blue color.
- Vasospasm? Pale color; try warm irrigation.
- Venous congestion? Wine stain (dark red color).

INTRAOPERATIVE NIPPLE–AREOLA COMPLEX PERFUSION EVALUATION

- Clinical judgment.
- Surgical instrument pressure/capillary refill monitoring (Video 2).
- Abrading the edge of incision with gauze to check bleeding.
- Warm irrigation to improve vasospasm.
- Blood pressure elevation.
- Indocyanine green dye via intravenous injection (Spy Elite technology, Novadaq, Bonita Springs, FL; see **Fig. 5**).

INTRAOPERATIVE NIPPLE–AREOLA COMPLEX REPERFUSION MANEUVERS

- Release sutures or tension at suture line.
- Relieve excessive kink/flexure of the pedicle.
- Evacuate hematoma, if present.
- Removal of implant, if present.
- Warm water irrigation.
- Blood pressure elevation.

POOR NIPPLE VASCULARITY

A pale or bluish NAC with limited bleeding on the cut edges needs very close postoperative observation. Poor or dark blue blood flow from the deepithelialized dermis is also a suspicious sign.[14,29] In these cases, Nitro-Bid cream can be applied to attempt vasodilatation. Patient rewarming and a normal blood pressure can reverse the changes associated with poor vascularity of the NAC that has originated owing to vasospasm; in these cases, perfusion will improve with normal capillary refill within the first hour after the end of the surgery.[30,31]

If, at the end of the surgery and after ensuring absence of hematoma, malrotation, and kinking of the pedicle, the situation does not improve, the NAC should be released from its inset position, effectively relieving tension on the NAC pedicle. The NAC will generally retract 1 or 2 cm, and if excessive suture tension of the NAC is the original cause, reperfusion will be noticed; if no immediate signs of NAC vitality are observed, the patient should be taken back to the operating room

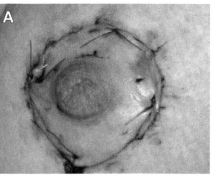
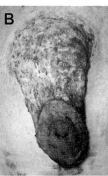
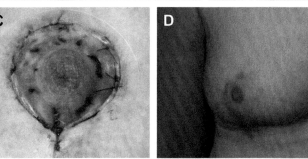

Fig. 5. (A–C) Nipple–areola complex suffering detected after surgery. Suture release was performed and resutured 3 days after with good result. (D) At 1 year postoperatively.

for conversion to a free NAC graft to a well-vascularized bed.[32,33] In this scenario, removing the NAC from its position on the pedicle and re-secting the distal portion of the pedicle is the suggested maneuver. The NAC is then applied as a full-thickness graft over the vital dermis as a "free nipple graft" (**Fig. 6**). If the nipple shows signs of ischemia in the early postoperative period (within 6 hours) despite normal blood pressure and core body temperature, a free graft must be undertaken immediately.[3] In some cases, NAC sufferance may not be identified in the early postoperative period and is detected too late to graft.[34] In these cases, conservative wound care is indicated, and secondary healing is the best option. NAC reconstruction is then undertaken at an appropriate time (usually 1 year after surgery), if needed.

FREE NIPPLE–AREOLA COMPLEX GRAFT INDICATIONS

For extremely large (>2000 g) reductions and very ptotic breasts with very long nipple to notch distances, a reliable pedicle to the NAC cannot always be preserved.[35] In these patients, an amputation is performed based on the Wise skin pattern, and the nipple is preserved and

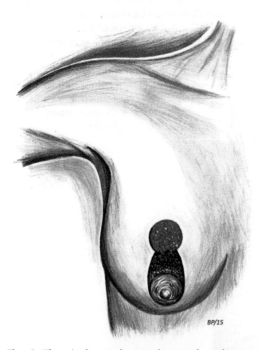

Fig. 6. The nipple–areola complex can be taken and grafted over the superior vital dermis portion of pedicle; the distal, nonvital portion of the pedicle must be resected.

repositioned as a free graft on a deepithelized bed. This is a safe and effective procedure for extremely large breasts and a less risky option for smokers. The nipple often undergoes desquamation in the course of healing, leading to partial pigment loss or loss of projection[36] (**Fig. 7**). A free NAC must be grafted to healthy deepithelialized vascularized dermis. Grafting to fat or to a poorly vascularized area will not work.

WHEN TO THINK ABOUT A FREE NIPPLE–AREOLA COMPLEX GRAFT

- Fear of nipple necrosis.
- Length pedicle (>10 cm mobilization).
- Large reductions (>2000 g).
- Severe ptosis, SN-N 35 cm.
- Very huge reductions, almost all breast amputations, usually in aging women, who suffer from related pain and discomfort.
- Patients with augmented risk factors.

COMPLICATIONS OF FREE NIPPLE GRAFTING

- Loss of ability to lactate.
- Loss of sensation.
- Loss of erectability.
- Loss of nipple projection.
- Possible hypopigmentation in dark-skinned patients.
- Possible nontake or partial "graft take.
- Poor cosmetic result.

POSTOPERATIVE CONTROL: HYPOTHERMIA AND PAIN

Adequate pain and postoperative body temperature control can improve cutaneous perfusion, and potentially improve healing.[16,33]

- Hypothermia induces peripheral vasoconstriction.[7,15]
- Painful stimuli cause a diffuse adrenergic discharge leading to cutaneous vasoconstriction.[8,16]

NECROTIC WOUND MANAGEMENT

In the case of more than 8 hours of NAC ischemia, consider it as an established damage. In this scenario, wound care management can be done mechanically, enzymatically, or surgically. Nonvital tissue must be removed, and the changing dressings twice a day is recommended to reduce bacterial contamination and promote quick granulation and reepithelialization (**Fig. 8**). We suggest the following course of treatment.

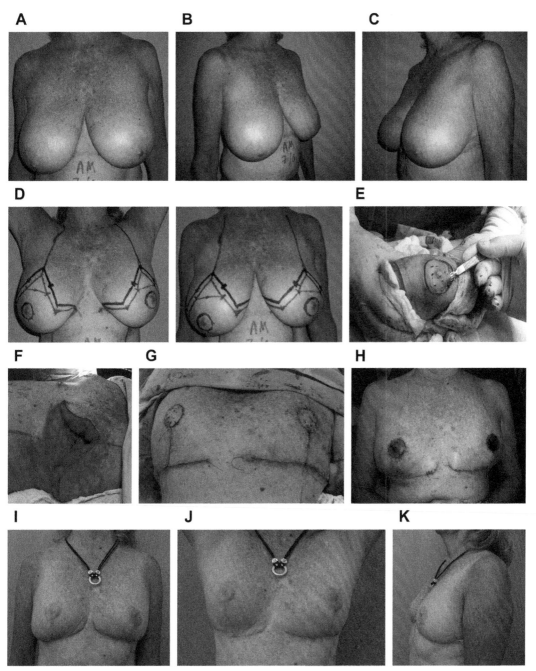

Fig. 7. (*A–C*) A 65-year-old woman who decided to make a huge reduction, front and lateral view. (*D*) Inverted T marking. (*E*) Taking the nipple–areola complex (NAC) graft. (*F*) Intraoperative view. Reduction. (*G*) Immediate result after NAC grafting. (*H*) At 1 week postoperatively. (*I–L*) At 1 year postoperatively, front and lateral views.

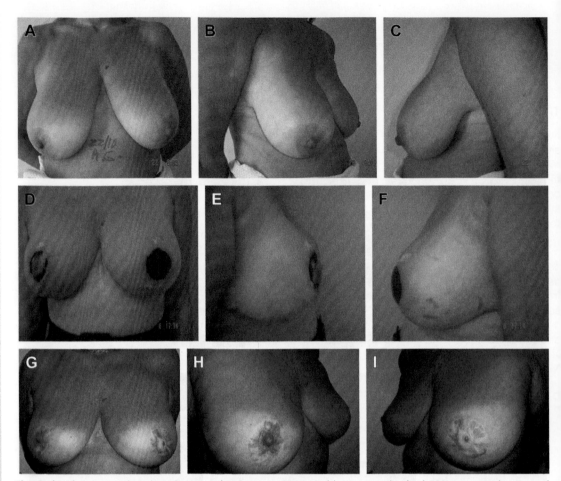

Fig. 8. (*A–C*) Preoperative view. Breast reduction in a 50-year-old woman who had 500 g resected over each breast with an inverted T. Superior internal pedicle. The patient was a heavy smoker. (*D–F*) Immediately Postoperatively. (*G–I*) At 2 years postoperatively. Conservative treatment was undertaken (wound care).

Initial Treatment

First 30 days

- Close personal contact with patient.
- Silver iron cream dressings with Atb.
- Surgical wound debridement of nonviable surrounding tissues.
- Autolytic agents, Iruxol N or collagenase creams.

After Debridement of All Necrotic Tissue

After 30 days

- Personal office follow-up, with weekly picture documentation in chart.
- Protease modulating agents, that is, Hydrogel and Alginate cream (moist environment to speed healing).

CAN WE PREDICT NIPPLE–AREOLA COMPLEX VIABILITY?

An objective assessment of blood flow to the nipple is done with the use of the indocyanine green dye, by intravenous injection. It is a useful way to assess tissue perfusion and vitality (Spy Elite technology). If there is confirmation of compromised NAC vascularity during surgery or within the first 6 hours postoperatively, an immediate free nipple graft should be performed.

INTRAOPERATIVE PROCEDURE TO CHECK TISSUE PERFUSION WITH INDOCYANINE GREEN

- Administer a 10-mg indocyanine green intravenously (12.5 mg in obese patients) rapid bolus.

- Administer a 10-mL saline rapid flush.
- Wait 8 to 10 seconds for circulation.
- Scan for 2 to 3 minutes.
- Analyze image.
- Repeat as desired during the procedure.

TREATMENT OF SEQUELAE

NAC ischemia does not always end favorably, and sequelae must be treated with proper patient information and consent. Depigmentation can be treated with tattooing, but the results vary and can be weak. Total nipple loss may require reconstruction with skin grafts and/or local flaps, tattoos, or with synthetic materials.

Bad scarring can alter NAC borders, and asymmetries produced by hypopigmentation are noticeable (**Fig. 9**), especially in dark-skinned patients. Tattooing scars can be a difficult task, and frequently it has to be repeated.[7,37] Sometimes, scars must be resected, and NAC resuturing is needed. The interlocking suture[15] has been demonstrated to be a good and practical maneuver as it maintains uniform tension around the NAC.

Different Available Options

- Intradermal tattoo.
- Nipple reconstruction with different pull-up flaps.
- These can be performed as ambulatory surgical procedures under local anesthesia and in an office setting. We usually recommend waiting at least 2 months between the nipple reconstruction and the areolar tattoo. In the

meantime, synthetic NAC reconstruction can be performed (**Figs. 10** and **11**).

SUMMARY

Even with a meticulous design, planning, and execution, 100% prevention of NAC ischemia and necrosis is not possible. NAC loss is a potential complication in every mammaplasty procedure and must be mentioned to patients, because it is not so rare as assumed. The assessment of the viability of a pedicled NAC after reduction mammaplasty can be frustrating owing to equivocal clinical signs of adequate blood supply.[38,39] NAC ischemia or NAC loss after breast reduction is a stressful situation for both the patient and the surgeon. Our suggestion for the appropriate action to be undertaken when this complication is detected varies depending on the time of detection:

- Intraoperative,
- Immediate postoperative (first 6 hours), or
- More than 6 hours postoperatively.

For the first 2 periods, active maneuvers have been described. After that, our suggestion is to wait and resect dead tissue and treat possible infection, allowing healing by secondary intention. It is this author's opinion that conservative management of full-thickness NAC loss may have a good cosmetic result, and in some cases, treatment of sequelae may not be required. It is important to recognize NAC ischemia on the operating table to take immediate corrective action and prevent necrosis when possible, but this is not always an easy task. If the postoperative evaluation is unclear,

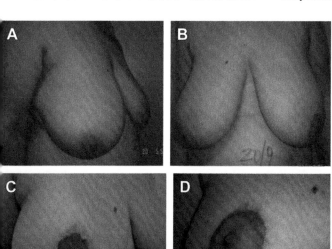

Fig. 9. (*A, B*) Preoperative photos: esthetic breast reduction. (*C, D*) Depigmented areolar borders and tattoo.

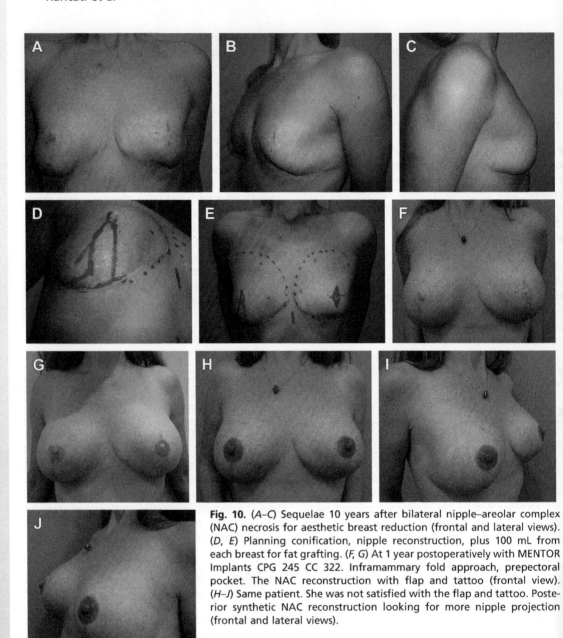

Fig. 10. (*A–C*) Sequelae 10 years after bilateral nipple–areolar complex (NAC) necrosis for aesthetic breast reduction (frontal and lateral views). (*D, E*) Planning conification, nipple reconstruction, plus 100 mL from each breast for fat grafting. (*F, G*) At 1 year postoperatively with MENTOR Implants CPG 245 CC 322. Inframammary fold approach, prepectoral pocket. The NAC reconstruction with flap and tattoo (frontal view). (*H–J*) Same patient. She was not satisfied with the flap and tattoo. Posterior synthetic NAC reconstruction looking for more nipple projection (frontal and lateral views).

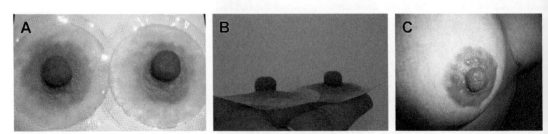

Fig. 11. (*A–C*) Synthetic nipple–areolar complex (NAC) of patient in **Fig. 10** by Naturally Impressive, LLC (Eau Claire, WI; frontal, lateral, and close up views).

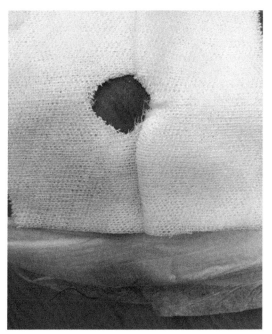

Fig. 12. Nipple monitor window dressing for immediate postoperatively.

later monitoring of NAC vitality is suggested within the first 6 hours postoperatively. This ensures that prompt and effective action is taken, if necessary. A dressing with a nipple monitor window is useful for this purpose (**Fig. 12**). Nipple areolar ischemia/necrosis is a real possibility in every mammaplasty procedure and must be mentioned in every mammaplasty informed consent form.

SUPPLEMENTARY DATA

Supplementary data related to this article can be found at http://dx.doi.org/10.1016/j.cps.2015.12.011.

REFERENCES

1. Grotting JC, Neligan PC, Beek AV, editors. Plastic surgery: breast. vol. 5. United Kingdom: Elsevier Health Science; 2012. p. 247.
2. Findlay EH. Ischemia of the nipple, areola, and skin flaps. In: Fisher J, Handel N, editors. Problems in breast surgery: a repair manual. CRC press; 2014. p. 493–5.
3. Wray RC, Luce EA. Treatment of impending nipple necrosis following reduction mammoplasty. Plast Reconstr Surg 1981;68:242–4.
4. van Deventer PV, Page BJ, Graewe FR. The safety of pedicles in breast reduction and mastopexy procedures. Aesthetic Plast Surg 2008;32:307–12.
5. Colombo G, Garlaschi A, Stifanese R, et al. Necrosis of the nipple areola complex, our personal way to solve problem. Ann Ital Chir 2015;86:156–62.
6. Penn J. FRCS breast reduction. Br J Plast Surg 1954;7:357–71.
7. Steed DL. Debridement. Am J Surg 2004;187:71S–4S.
8. Corduff N, Rozen WM, Taylor GI. The superficial venous drainage of the breast: a clinical study and implications for breast reduction surgery. J Plast Reconstr Aesthet Surg 2010;63:809–13.
9. Masia J, Larranaga J, Clavero JA, et al. The value of the multidetector row computed tomography for the preoperative planning of deep inferior epigastric artery perforator flap: our experience in 162 cases. Ann Plast Surg 2008;60:29–36.
10. Craig RD, Sykes PA. Nipple sensitivity following reduction mammoplasty. Br J Plast Surg 1970;23:165–72.
11. Bernard T, Lee BT. Impact of complications on patient satisfaction in breast reconstruction. Plast Reconstr Surg 2011;127:1428.
12. Nahai F, Nahai F. Breast reduction. Plast Reconstr Surg 2008;121:1.
13. Mojallal A, Comparin JP, Voulliaume D, et al. Reduction mammaplasty using superior pedicle in macromastia. Ann Chir Plast Esthet 2005;50:118–26.
14. Manahan MA, Buretta KJ, Chang D, et al. An outcomes analysis of 2142 breast reduction procedures. Ann Plast Surg 2015;74:289–92.
15. Hammond DH. Short-scar periareolar inferior pedicle reduction SPAIR mammaplasty. In: Operative techniques in plastic and reconstructive surgery. Elsevier; 2009. p. 106–18.
16. Lugo LM, Prada M, Kohanzadeh S, et al. Surgical outcomes of gigantomastia breast reduction superomedial pedicle technique: a 12-year retrospective study. Ann Plast Surg 2013;70:533–7.
17. Stolier AJ, Levine EA. Reducing the risk of nipple necrosis: technical observations in 340 nipple-sparing mastectomies. Breast J 2013;19:173–9.
18. le Roux CM, Pan WR, Matousek SA, et al. Preventing venous congestion of the nipple-areola complex: an anatomical guide to preserving essential venous drainage networks. Plast Reconstr Surg 2011;127:1073–9.
19. Hofmann AK, Wuestner-Hofmann MC, Bassetto F, et al. Breast reduction: modified "Lejour technique" in 500 large breasts. Plast Reconstr Surg 2007;120:1095–104 [discussion: 1105–7].
20. Lypka M, Rizvi M, Lapuerta L. The Graf/Biggs flap to increase upper pole projection in breast reductions with free nipple grafts. Aesthetic Plast Surg 2010;34:687–90.
21. Landau AG, Hudson DA. Choosing the superomedial pedicle for reduction mammaplasty in gigantomastia. Plast Reconstr Surg 2008;121:735–9.

22. Spear SL, Rottman SJ, Seiboth LA, et al. Breast reconstruction using a staged nipple-sparing mastectomy following mastopexy or reduction. Plast Reconstr Surg 2012;129:572–81.

23. O'Dey DM, Prescher A, Pallua N. Vascular reliability of nipple-areola complex-bearing pedicles: an anatomical microdissection study. Plast Reconstr Surg 2006;118:292–3.

24. Wrye SW, Banducci DR, Mackay D, et al. Routine drainage is not required in reduction mammaplasty. Plast Reconstr Surg 2003;111:113–7.

25. Nahabedian MY, Mofid MM. Viability and sensation of the nipple-areolar complex after reduction mammaplasty. Ann Plast Surg 2002;49:24–31 [discussion: 31–2].

26. Roth AC, Zook EG, Brown R, et al. Nipple-areolar perfusion and reduction mammaplasty: correlation of laser Doppler readings with surgical complications. Plast Reconstr Surg 1996;97:381–6.

27. Hallock GG. Salvage by tattooing of areolar complications following breast reduction. Plast Reconstr Surg 1993;91:942–5.

28. Wang P, Nuveen EJ. Diagnosis and management of areolar ischemia. Am J Cosmet Surg 2012;29(2):159–70.

29. Cunningham L. The anatomy of the arteries and veins of the breast. J Surg Oncol 1977;9:71–85.

30. Hester TR Jr, Bostwick J 3rd, Miller L, et al. Breast reduction utilizing the maximally vascularized central breast pedicle. Plast Reconstr Surg 1985;76:890–900.

31. Wuringer E, Mader N, Posch E, et al. Nerve and vessel sup- plying ligamentous suspension of the mammary gland. Plast Reconstr Surg 1998;101:1486–93.

32. Wueringer E, Tschabitscher M. New aspects of the topographical anatomy of the mammary gland regarding its neurovascular supply along a regular ligamentous suspension. Eur J Morphol 2002;40:181–9.

33. Gates JL, Holloway GA. A comparison of wound environments. Ostomy Wound Manage 1992;38:34–7.

34. Hallock GG, Cusenz BJ. Aesthetic salvage of the congested nipple during reduction mammoplasty. Aesthetic Plast Surg 1986;10:143–5.

35. Foster L, Moore P. Acute surgical wound care. 3: fitting the dressing to the wound. Br J Nurs 1999;8:204, 206.

36. Cutting K, White R, Hoekstra H. Topical silver-impregnated dressings and the importance of the dressing technology. Int Wound J 2009;6:396–402.

37. Ramundo J, Gray M. Collagenase for enzymatic debridement: a systematic review. J Wound Ostomy Continence Nurs 2009;36(Suppl 6):S4–11.

38. Knig M, Vanscheidt W, Augustin M, et al. Enzymatic versus autolytic debridement of chronic leg ulcers: a prospective randomised trial. J Wound Care 2005;14:320–3.

39. Woods JE, Meland NB. Conservative management in full-thickness nipple-areolar necrosis after subcutaneous mastectomy. Plast Reconstr Surg 1989;84:258–64 [discussion: 265–6].

Managing Necrosis of the Nipple Areolar Complex Following Reduction Mammaplasty and Mastopexy

Neal Handel, MD*, Sara Yegiyants, MD

KEYWORDS

- NAC necrosis • Reduction mammaplasty • Reduction mastopexy • Prevention • Management
- Reconstruction of ischemic necrosis of NAC

KEY POINTS

- Necrosis of the nipple areolar complex (NAC) is an infrequent but devastating complication of reduction mammaplasty and mastopexy. However, with strategic management and properly timed reconstruction, it is possible in most cases to restore a natural-appearing NAC.
- To prevent necrosis of the NAC, it is most important to maintain a pedicle of adequate thickness, be cognizant of the length to width ratio of the pedicle, prevent kinking the blood supply when insetting the flap, and avoid an excessively tight skin closure, no matter what type of technique is performed. Especially in the case of secondary reduction mammaplasty or mastopexy in the previously augmented patient, great care must be taken because the breast anatomy and physiology has changed because of the previous procedures.
- In the immediate postoperative period, the ischemic NAC can be transferred as a full-thickness graft. When it is elected to convert to a graft, all the circulatory changes have to be stabilized to confirm that the ischemia is irreversible and the recipient site is healthy enough to accept a graft.
- The guiding principle in surgical management of ischemic complications of the NAC is to avoid aggressive treatment until the tissue necrosis obviously demarcates. When the missing part is small, the nipple can be reconstructed by composite grafting from the contralateral nipple. When a major part of the nipple is lost, reconstruction using a local flap can yield a favorable result.
- The areola can be reconstructed using a full skin graft from the contralateral areola, the labia minora, or the upper inner thigh. Intradermal tattooing can be used to obtain a desirable color match.

INTRODUCTION

Necrosis of the nipple areolar complex (NAC) is an infrequent but dreaded complication of reduction mammaplasty and mastopexy. When there is significant loss of nipple and/or areolar tissue, it not only results in major cosmetic deformity but also may be a source of great angst for the surgeon and patients alike.

The manifestations of nipple areolar ischemia run the gamut from spontaneous, completely reversible nipple congestion (**Fig. 1**) to total loss

Division of Plastic Surgery, Geffen School of Medicine at University of California Los Angeles, Los Angeles, CA, USA
* Corresponding author. 22 West Pueblo Street, Suite A, Santa Barbara, CA 93105.
E-mail address: nh@drhandel.com

Clin Plastic Surg 43 (2016) 415–423
http://dx.doi.org/10.1016/j.cps.2015.12.012
0094-1298/16/$ – see front matter © 2016 Elsevier Inc. All rights reserved.

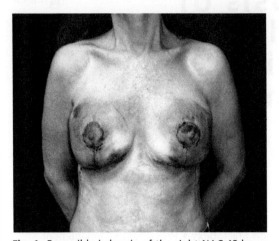

Fig. 1. Reversible ischemia of the right NAC 48 hours after reduction mammaplasty.

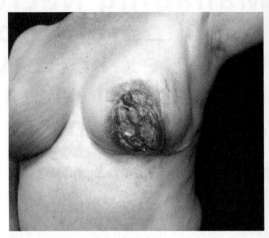

Fig. 3. Total loss of the NAC and extensive fat necrosis of subadjacent breast tissue.

of the nipple (**Fig. 2**) with extensive necrosis of subadjacent breast tissue (**Fig. 3**). The appropriate response to nipple ischemia depends on the degree of circulatory compromise. The guiding principle is to avoid aggressive surgical therapy as long as possible to give the injured tissues the best possible chance to recover spontaneously.

Circulatory compromise of the NAC may be due to arterial insufficiency but is more commonly caused by venous congestion.[1] Clinical signs of venous congestion include excessively brisk capillary refill, dark rapid bleeding on pinprick, and cyanosis and edema of the nipple. Venous congestion can occur for a variety of reasons: inadequate preservation of venous drainage, long pedicles, kinking or compression of the pedicle, excessively tight skin closure, or a hematoma.

The risk of nipple areolar ischemia is increased with large-volume tissue removal, transposition of the NAC a great distance (more than 15 cm),[2] and in cases whereby secondary mastopexy is performed in previously augmented patients.[3] Systemic factors, such as obesity, diabetes, and cigarette smoking, may also increase the risk of ischemia.

The objectives of this article are to explain the mechanisms of injury that result in ischemia of the NAC, to offer recommendations about the management of this complication, and to illustrate reconstructive techniques that can be used to correct deformities arising from necrosis of the NAC. With these goals in mind, the remainder of this article is divided into 3 sections: (1) prevention of ischemia of the NAC, (2) management of the ischemic nipple, and (3) reconstruction after ischemic necrosis of the nipple and areola.

PREVENTING ISCHEMIA OF THE NIPPLE AREOLAR COMPLEX

Clearly, preventing ischemic complications is greatly preferable to treating a necrotic nipple and areola. When performing reduction mammaplasty or mastopexy, care must be taken to select the operation that will likely produce the best outcome with the least risk of complications.

Understanding of breast vascular anatomy is crucial in preserving the arterial inflow and the essential venous drainage network of the nipple areola complex. Cadaveric dissection studies have shown that the most reliable blood supply to the nipple areola complex is from the internal thoracic–anterior intercostal system, supplying the NAC from the medio-inferior aspect. An

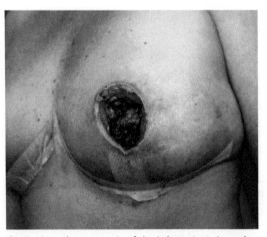

Fig. 2. Complete necrosis of the left NAC 10 days after reduction mammaplasty.

additional collateral system composed of lateral thoracic and other minor contributors supplies the NAC from the superolateral aspect.[1] Venograms of the breast have shown an extensive network of veins draining the NAC with the most reliable patterns located in the superomedial/medial and inferior pedicles.[4]

A wide variety of techniques have been described for transferring the nipple in breast reduction and mastopexy. The most commonly performed procedure combines the Wise-pattern skin incision with an inferior pedicle for nipple transposition. This operation has gained popularity because of the reliability of the blood supply to the nipple, the relatively short learning curve, and the applicability of this method to reductions of all sizes. The main drawback to this approach is that aesthetic results are not always optimal. There may be a boxy contour to the breasts; it can be difficult to achieve desired breast projection; there is a tendency to pseudoptosis over time; and there is invariably a long scar in the inframammary fold. For these reasons, a variety of alternate pedicles and different skin patterns have evolved. In addition to the traditional inferior pedicle, the superior, superomedial, and central pedicle have all been successfully used in breast reduction and mastopexy. The reported rates of nipple necrosis vary with the use of different pedicles ranging from 0.8 % to 2.3% (0.8% with inferior pedicle, 2.1% total nipple necrosis with the use of superodermal pedicle, and 2.3% with superolateral pedicle).[1] However, there are no randomized controlled trials comparing NAC necrosis rates for the different techniques.

In recent years, short scar techniques, including the vertical pattern[5] and short-scar periareolar-inferior pedicle reduction (SPAIR) technique,[6] have been introduced. Because there are so many possible combinations and permutations of skin pattern and vascular pedicle, it is difficult to objectively compare one technique with another. In a recent matched cohort study,[7] the investigators compared superomedial pedicle vertical scar breast reduction with inferior pedicle Wise-pattern reduction and found there was no significant difference in complications between these two techniques. It is likely that adherence to the basic principles of plastic surgery is more critical than the particular surgical technique selected. Regardless of which approach is chosen, the surgeon must be careful to maintain a pedicle of adequate thickness, be cognizant of the length to width ratio of the pedicle, prevent kinking the blood supply when insetting the flap, and avoid excessively tight skin closure.

One group of patients especially at risk for ischemic complications of the NAC is previously augmented women with ptosis who present for mastopexy. These patients are at increased risk of circulatory compromise because of the inevitable changes in breast anatomy and physiology caused by implants. In many augmented patients, the soft-tissue envelope surrounding the implant becomes attenuated. Tebbetts[8] observed: "The consequences of excessively large breast implants include ptosis, tissue stretching, tissue thinning, inadequate soft-tissue cover, [and] subcutaneous tissue atrophy." These very same changes occur not just with "excessively large" implants as described by Tebbetts but with all breast implants to some degree over time. Most of the thinning and atrophy caused by implants occurs in the inferior pole of the breast. It is important to take this into account when selecting which pedicle to use in patients undergoing secondary mastopexy. A conventional Wise-pattern skin excision coupled with an inferior pedicle may be prone to ischemia because of thinning of the tissues of the inferior pole. In such cases, it may be prudent to preserve a superior pedicle as well (as in a traditional McKissock reduction mammaplasty) to ensure adequate arterial perfusion and sufficient venous drainage. Vertical mastopexy techniques are applicable in previously augmented patients; however, vertical techniques that depend on an inferior pedicle, such as the SPAIR mammaplasty may be relatively contraindicated. Procedures that incorporate a superior pedicle (Lejour, Lassus, Hall-Findlay) are probably safer in terms of preserving circulation to the nipple and areola.

When selecting the specific mastopexy operation for correction ptosis in augmented patients, there is a wide spectrum of procedures from which to choose. These procedures include crescent nipple lift, periareolar mastopexy, vertical lift, and finally the conventional Wise-pattern mastopexy. In general, the least aggressive mastopexy that will achieve the desired result is preferred. In secondary mastopexy patients, it is also critical to consider the effect of prior skin incisions on the blood supply of the nipple and the skin flaps and to avoid insertion of excessively large implants, which may cause compression of the vascular pedicle and lead to venous congestion.

MANAGING ISCHEMIA OF THE NIPPLE AREOLAR COMPLEX

When circulatory compromise of the nipple and areola is recognized early, either in the operating room or in the immediate postoperative period, urgent steps should be undertaken to reduce permanent tissue loss. Recognition of irreversible ischemia of the nipple may be hard to determine by clinical criteria alone. Intravenous fluorescein has been used to assess viability of the nipple.[9] Indocyanine green videofluorography[10] is a newer technique that can be used to evaluate NAC viability intraoperatively. Advantages of this technique include repeated use during the same operation and ability to evaluate both the arterial microcirculation and venous outflow. Intraoperative detection of NAC nonviability is an indication to convert to a full-thickness graft. In cases whereby there is irreversible ischemia of the nipple, conversion of the nipple from a pedicle flap to a full-thickness graft can result in a satisfactory aesthetic outcome.[11] However, before making the decision to convert the nipple to a full-thickness graft, it is prudent to wait until the circulatory changes related to tissue cooling and the intraoperative use of epinephrine have subsided. If it is elected to convert to a graft, it is crucial that the recipient site have an excellent blood supply. This requirement precludes grafting onto breast tissue or fat; the graft must be affixed to a healthy dermal bed.

Conversion of the nipple to a graft is indicated only rarely and in dire cases. In most circumstances whereby ischemia of the nipple is identified early, conservative measures are effective in reversing or at least ameliorating the problem

(**Fig. 4**). Release of the dermal and subdermal sutures around the periphery of the areola may result in dramatic improvement in venous drainage with transformation of tissues from a violaceous hue to a pink color within a matter of minutes. The application of Nitroglycerin Ointment USP, 2% (Nitro-Bid) may help by causing vasodilation and promoting drainage of blood. Steroids, such as a methylprednisolone (Medrol Dosepak), have also been recommended to reduce local tissue swelling and promote venous drainage. Leeches can also be used to improve venous drainage.[12] Consideration should also be given to the use of hyperbaric oxygen therapy.[13] The mechanism of action of hyperbaric oxygen therapy is to increase tissue oxygen tension, which results in production of reactive oxygen species and reactive nitrogen species that promote neovascularization and improve postischemic tissue survival.[14]

The guiding principle in surgical management of ischemic complications of the NAC is to avoid aggressive treatment until the tissues have declared themselves. It is often difficult early in the acute phase to gauge which tissues will ultimately prove viable and which tissues will necrose (**Fig. 5A–L**). During the interim it is advisable to maintain patients on oral antibiotics to reduce the risk of infection. A wide variety of antimicrobials are available and include drugs such as penicillin VK 500 mg every 6 hours or cephalexin 500 mg

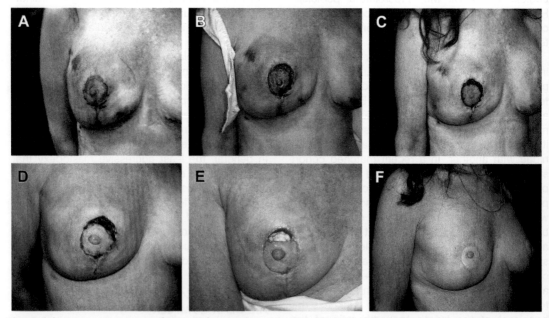

Fig. 4. (A) Venous congestion of NAC 48 hours after reduction mammaplasty; (B) appearance of NAC 72 hours after removal of skin and subdermal sutures; (C) improved appearance of NAC at POD No. 7; (D) further improvement in circulation at POD No. 10; (E) fat necrosis of underlying breast tissue treated by surgical debridement and delayed primary closure; (F) appearance 18 months after procedure.

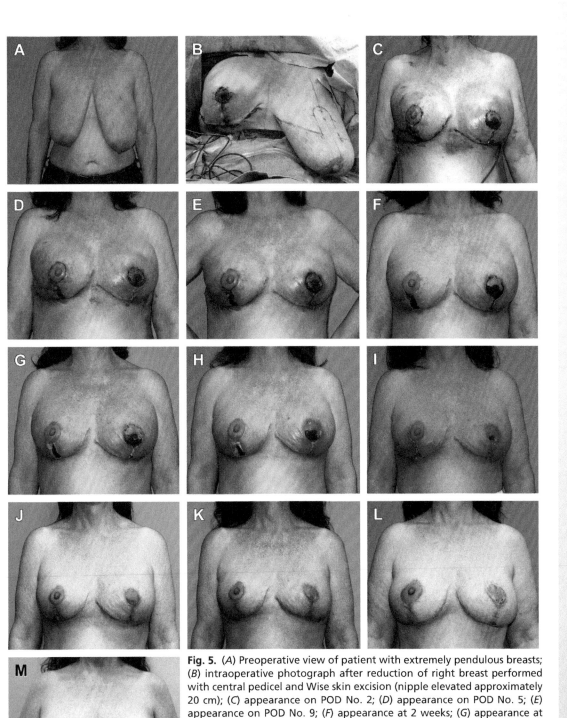

Fig. 5. (A) Preoperative view of patient with extremely pendulous breasts; (B) intraoperative photograph after reduction of right breast performed with central pedicel and Wise skin excision (nipple elevated approximately 20 cm); (C) appearance on POD No. 2; (D) appearance on POD No. 5; (E) appearance on POD No. 9; (F) appearance at 2 weeks; (G) appearance at 3 weeks; (H) appearance at 5 weeks; (I) appearance at 2 months; (J) appearance at 3 months; (K) appearance at 4 months; (L) appearance at 2 years: patient was offered further reconstruction of left NAC but declined additional surgery; (M) appearance at 7 years without reconstruction.

every 6 hours. Consideration should be given to adding trimethoprim and sulfamethoxazole (Bactrim DS) twice a day to the regimen as prophylaxis against methicillin-resistant *Staphylococcus* *aureus*. In addition to systemic antibiotics, topical antimicrobials may be used to further reduce the chance of secondary infection. Several topical agents are commonly used for this purpose, such

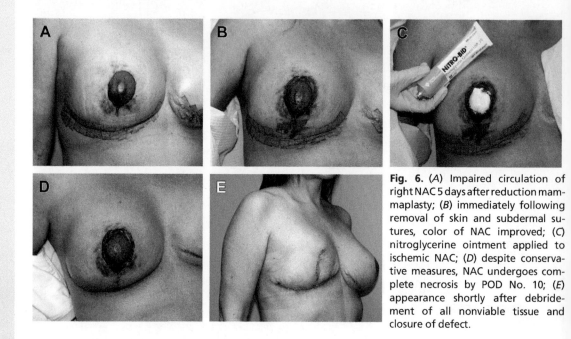

Fig. 6. (*A*) Impaired circulation of right NAC 5 days after reduction mammaplasty; (*B*) immediately following removal of skin and subdermal sutures, color of NAC improved; (*C*) nitroglycerine ointment applied to ischemic NAC; (*D*) despite conservative measures, NAC undergoes complete necrosis by POD No. 10; (*E*) appearance shortly after debridement of all nonviable tissue and closure of defect.

as neomycin-polymyxin B-bacitracin (Neosporin) triple antibiotic ointment or 1% silver sulfadiazine (Silvadene cream).

Once the tissues have demarcated and it is clear how much of the NAC will survive and how much is necrotic, a decision can be made about appropriate surgical management. If the area of nonviable tissue is limited (partial loss of nipple, subtotal loss of areola), allowing the necrotic tissues to slough and the resulting defect to heal by secondary intention may be the most prudent approach. If the amount of necrotic tissue is more sizable, debridement and delayed primary closure may be indicated (**Fig. 6**). Regardless of whether the defect is allowed to close spontaneously or is closed surgically, there should be a delay before any reconstructive procedure is

attempted. It is critical to give the injured tissues time to recover before proceeding with further intervention. A waiting period of 3 to 6 months is usually adequate to allow for resolution of inflammation, improvement in local circulation, and maturation and softening of scar tissue.

RECONSTRUCTION OF THE NECROTIC NIPPLE AND AREOLA

After a suitable waiting period has transpired, reconstruction of the defect may commence. The appropriate reconstructive procedure depends on the nature of the deficit. In some cases, the amount of missing tissue is negligible, which facilitates reconstruction. For example, if only a portion of the areola is absent, it may be possible to

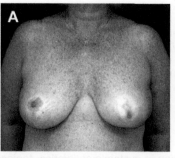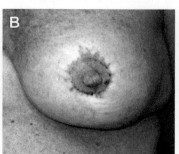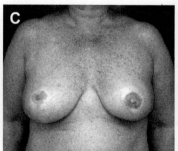

Fig. 7. (*A*) Patient referred for reconstruction of left NAC lost following reduction mammaplasty; (*B*) appearance of reconstructed NAC 3 weeks after procedure, nipple was reconstructed with a modified skate flap and areola from full-thickness skin graft from upper inner thigh; (*C*) appearance 1 year following reconstruction, there has been some loss of projection of the reconstructed nipple, which is typical in these cases.

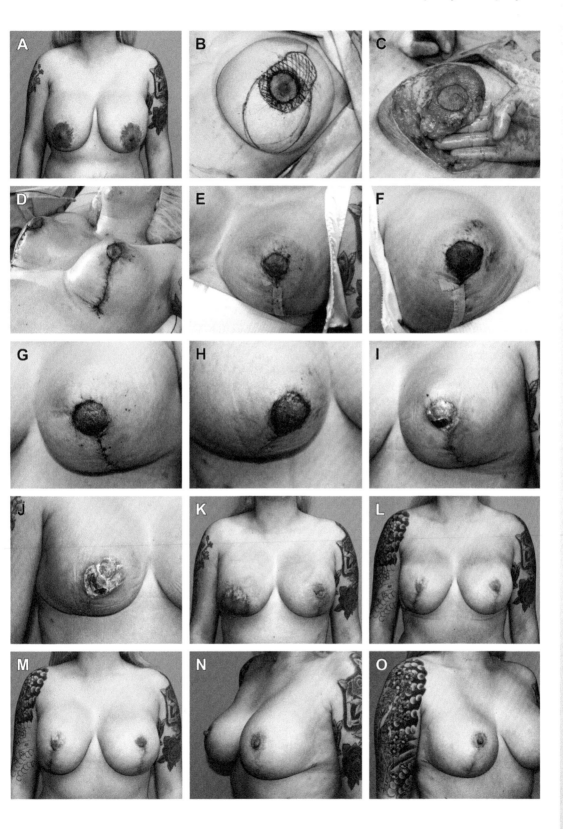

reconstruct the defect with a full-thickness graft from the contralateral areola. Likewise, if the areola is intact but part or even the entire nipple has been lost, a composite graft from the opposite nipple may be indicated (assuming there is adequate tissue for sharing). In some cases there is residual nipple and/or areola, but the degree of tissue damage or tissue loss is so extensive that the best approach is to discard the remaining tissue and perform de novo nipple areolar reconstruction. In such cases, or when the NAC has been completely lost, there are many excellent techniques for recreating a natural-appearing nipple.

A host of operations have been described for reconstruction of the mammary papilla or nipple. Composite grafts, such as the pulp of the toe[15] or the earlobe, have been used to reconstruct the missing nipple. However, even when these grafts take successfully, they do not match the texture or pigmentation of a normal nipple. Composite grafts from the contralateral nipple can yield an excellent aesthetic result provided there is adequate nipple on the intact side to serve as a donor site. More commonly, the papilla is reconstructed with local tissues. These procedures typically consist of some type of random flap, which is elevated and rotated or folded to create a projecting structure of the desired size and shape. Among the operations that have been described are the star flap,[16,17] the double opposing tab flap,[18] and the double opposing periareola flap.[19] Most of these techniques are derivatives of the skate flap,[20] which has proven to be a safe and reliable technique for reconstruction of the nipple.[21] The skate flap is popular because it is relatively easy to learn and results are predictable. The skate flap has a hardy blood supply, which ensures survival of the tissue and promotes maintenance of long-term projection of the reconstructed nipple (**Fig. 7**).

It is important to remember that reconstruction of the nipple in patients who have had ischemic necrosis of the native NAC differs substantially from reconstruction of the nipple in mastectomy patients. Unless mastectomy patients have been irradiated, the skin at the site of NAC reconstruction is generally in good condition; it is typically supple, unscarred, and has a good blood supply. This condition facilitates successful reconstruction of the nipple with any of a variety of local flaps and provides a well-vascularized recipient site for application of either full-thickness or composite grafts. Patients who have lost their NAC as a result of ischemic complications are more likely to have scarred, poorly vascularized tissues at the site of the proposed reconstruction. When planning nipple reconstruction, it is important to consider the quality of the local tissues in designing pedicles to ensure the best chance of flap survival (**Fig. 8**).

With regard to reconstruction of the areola, the most natural-appearing areola is created using a full-thickness skin graft from the contralateral breast. The feasibility of using the opposite areole as a donor site depends of course on how much tissue is available for harvesting. Fortunately, the areola tends to be a very elastic structure; if a washer-shaped piece of pigmented skin is harvested from the periphery of the intact areola, the residual pigmented skin will usually stretch enough so the donor areola maintains a reasonable size. Other sites that have been used for areolar reconstruction include full-thickness grafts from the labia minora and the upper inner thigh. Although the early results of these grafts are often very pleasing, there is a tendency for the grafted skin to lose pigmentation over time. Frequently after an interval of 2 to 3 years following reconstruction, the pigmentation has completely faded and the only indication of areolar reconstruction is a circular scar around the periphery of the

Fig. 8. (A) A 23-year-old woman who previously had bilateral augmentation mammaplasty and circumareolar mastopexy presents with dissatisfaction due to persistent breast ptosis and disfigured NACs; (B) design for vertical mastopexy with superior pedicle for transposition of nipple; (C) intraoperative view after nipple has been mobilized, note relatively short distance nipple needs to be raised and thick (3 cm) superior pedicle; (D) appearance of the breast at completion of procedure, both NACs appear viable; (E, F) appearance 4 days after procedure significant venous congestion of NACs, right side worse than left side, dermal sutures released, and nitroglycerine paste applied; (G, H) appearance 10 days after procedure, necrotic eschar separating revealing partial survival of areola bilaterally; (I, J) appearance 24 days after procedure, central band of tissue on left side has survived but only tiny amount of tissue on right side is viable; (K) 6 weeks after procedure, open areas characterized by healthy granulation tissue, and patient undergoes delayed primary closure of wounds bilaterally; (L) by 4 months after delayed closure, both breast have healed; (M) at 6 months tissues have softened and scars have matured, and patient is ready for reconstruction; (N, O) 3 months following bilateral NAC reconstruction, nipple has been created using a modified skate flap with care taken to incorporate residual pigmented tissue into reconstructed papilla, and areolae have been reconstructed from full-thickness skin grafts from upper inner thigh.

reconstructed nipple. For this reason, intradermal tattooing has gained great popularity for areolar reconstruction. Tattooing can be used either with or without preliminary skin grafting.[22] The tattooed areola may also fade over time, but touch up tattooing is a relatively easy way to restore the desired pigmentation. When the nipple is reconstructed from local tissue (eg, skate flap or other local flap), it does not match the color of the intact contralateral nipple. Tattooing of the papilla is the easiest way to achieve the desired color match. Because symmetry is such an important component of successful nipple reconstruction, it may be advisable to also tattoo the intact NAC to achieve the best possible color match between the two sides.

Necrosis of all or part of the NAC after reduction mammaplasty or mastopexy is a devastating complication. It is not only disappointing for patients but can also be disheartening for the surgeon. However, with properly timed and well-executed reconstructive procedures, it is possible in most cases to restore a very natural-appearing NAC.

REFERENCES

1. van Deventer PV, Page BJ, Graewe FR. The safety of pedicles in breast reduction and mastopexy procedures. Aesthetic Plast Surg 2008;32:307–12.

2. Gravante G, Araco A, Sorge R, et al. Postoperative wound infections after breast reductions: the role of smoking and the amount of tissue removed. Aesthetic Plast Surg 2008;32:25–31.

3. Handel N. Secondary mastopexy in the augmented patient: a recipe for disaster. Plast Reconstr Surg 2006;118(7 Suppl):152S–63S.

4. le Roux CM, Pan WR, Matousek SA. Preventing venous congestion of the nipple-areola complex: an anatomical guide to preserving essential venous drainage networks. Plast Reconstr Surg 2011;127(3):1073–9.

5. Hall-Findlay EJ. Vertical breast reduction with a medially based pedicle. Aesthet Surg J 2002;22:185–94.

6. Hammond DC. Short scar periareolar inferior pedicle reduction (SPAIR) mammaplasty. Plast Reconstr Surg 1999;103:890–901.

7. Antony AK, Yegiyants SS, Danielson KK, et al. A matched cohort study of superomedial pedicle vertical scar breast reduction (100 breasts) and traditional inferior pedicle wise-pattern reduction (100 breasts): an outcomes study over 3 years. Plast Reconstr Surg 2013;132(5):1068–76.

8. Tebbetts JB. The greatest myths in breast augmentation. Plast Reconstr Surg 2001;107:1895–903.

9. Singer R, Krant SM. Intravenous fluorescein for evaluating the dusky nipple-areola during reduction mammaplasty. Plast Reconstr Surg 1981;67(4):534–5.

10. Murray JD, Jones GE, Elwood T. Fluorescent intraoperative tissue angiography with indocyanine green: evaluation of nipple-areola vascularity during breast reduction surgery. Plast Reconstr Surg 2010;126(1):33e–4e.

11. Wray RC, Luce EA. Treatment of impending nipple necrosis following reduction mammaplasty. Plast Reconstr Surg 1981;68(2):242–4.

12. Pannucci CJ, Nelson JA, Chung CU, et al. Medicinal leeches for surgically uncorrectable venous congestion after free flap breast reconstruction. Microsurgery 2014;34(7):522–6.

13. Friedman HI, Fitzmaurice M, Lefaivre JF, et al. An evidence-based appraisal of the use of hyperbaric oxygen on flaps and grafts. Plast Reconstr Surg 2006;117(7 Suppl):175S–90S.

14. Thom SR. Hyperbaric oxygen: its mechanisms and efficacy. Plast Reconstr Surg 2011;127(Suppl 1):131S–41S.

15. Klatsky SA, Manson PN. Toe pulp free grafts in nipple reconstruction. Plast Reconstr Surg 1981;68(2):245–8.

16. Sierakowski A, Niranjan N. Star flap with a dermal platform for nipple reconstruction. J Plast Reconstr Aesthet Surg 2011;64(2):e55–6.

17. Eskenazi L. A one-stage nipple reconstruction with the "modified star" flap and immediate tattoo: a review of 100 cases. Plast Reconstr Surg 1993;92(4):671–80.

18. Kroll SS, Reece GP, Miller MJ, et al. Comparison of nipple projection with the modified double-opposing tab and star flaps. Plast Reconstr Surg 1997;99:1602–5.

19. Shestak KC, Nguyen TD. The double opposing periareola flap: a novel concept for nipple-areola reconstruction. Plast Reconstr Surg 2007;119(2):473–80.

20. Little JW. Nipple areolar reconstruction. In: Cohen M, editor. Mastery of plastic and reconstructive surgery, vol. II. Boston: Little, Brown; 1994. p. 1342–8.

21. Hammond DC, Khuthaila D, Kim J. The skate flap purse-string technique for nipple-areola complex reconstruction. Plast Reconstr Surg 2007;120(2):399–406.

22. Becker H. The use of intradermal tattoo to enhance the final result of nipple-areola reconstruction. Plast Reconstr Surg 1986;77(4):673–5.

Breast Reduction in the Burned Breast

 CrossMark

Karen L. Powers, MD[a], Linda G. Phillips, MD[b],*

KEYWORDS

• Breast reduction • Burn • Burned breast • Mammaplasty

KEY POINTS

• Mammary hypertrophy can occur in the postburn breast, despite scarring and contractures; patients with burned breasts exhibit the same symptoms of symptomatic macromastia as patients with unburned breasts do.
• Although breast volume reduction is the ultimate goal, the contour of the breast must first be restored by releasing scar contractures.
• Regardless of the reduction mammaplasty technique used, the inelastic nature of grafted and scarred scar requires a conservative approach to tissue elevation and transposition.

INTRODUCTION

With improvements in burn care, patients survive increasingly large total body surface area (TBSA) burns. In a series of large TBSA burns, the breasts were the most frequently injured area within the trunk/perineal region.[1] McCauley and colleagues[2] noted that 71% of female patients with burns to the anterior chest wall with involvement of the nipple-areolar complex (NAC) will require surgical intervention. Mammary hypertrophy can occur in the postburn breast, despite scarring and contractures. Patients with burned breasts exhibit the same symptoms of symptomatic macromastia as patients with unburned breasts do. This condition may occur unilaterally in which a reduction mammaplasty may be required for symmetry with the burned breast. Alternately, bilateral reduction mammaplasties may be required if both breasts are hypertrophic.[3] Thai and colleagues[4] noted that, although many plastic surgeons are reluctant to operate on burned breasts for fear of devascularizing the skin graft or NAC, reduction mammaplasty in this group of patients is safe

and carries minimal risk if certain key concepts are followed.

RISKS OF OPERATING ON BURNED BREASTS

Early tangential excision of burns to the anterior chest wall is currently the standard of care. McCauley and colleagues[2] note, however, this approach is modified at many burn centers when dealing with the anterior chest wall burns in young female patients. In such cases, the eschar may be allowed to demarcate and separate before tangential excision; some surgeons mark the areas of the breast bud before surgical intervention in order to avoid destruction during debridement of more superficial burns. Such advancements in surgical technique avoid the risk of damaging a breast bud uninjured by the burn; in some patients this undamaged breast bud creates macromastia in the future.

Surgical manipulation of the hypertrophic burned breast comes with its own risks, including flap necrosis, poor wound healing, and poor aesthetic outcomes. As discussed later, a conservative stepwise approach is key.

Disclosure statement: The authors have nothing to disclose.
[a] Section of Plastic Surgery, Department of Surgery, Lakeland Regional Medical Center, St. Joseph, MI, USA;
[b] Division of Plastic Surgery, Department of Surgery, University of Texas Medical Branch, 301 University Boulevard, Galveston, TX 77555-0724, USA
* Corresponding author.
E-mail address: lphillip@utmb.edu

plasticsurgery.theclinics.com

EVALUATION OF THE HYPERTROPHIC BURNED BREAST

Several factors are assessed preoperatively to evaluate the extent of the damage and its effect on mammary hypertrophy. Just as McCauley and colleagues[2] note in reconstruction of the burned breast, the extent of the deformity, the location of the deformity, and the status of the surrounding soft tissue are all assessed before embarking on any surgical plan. Scar contractures can be detected early, particularly when an uninjured breast serves as a landmark for distortions in shape or NAC position. Deformity of a hypertrophic breast is addressed separately from deformities of the inframammary region alone.

PRINCIPLES FOR REDUCING THE BURNED BREAST
Improve Breast Contour by Releasing Scar Contractures

Completely release breast tissue distorted secondary to burns through either incision or excision of burn scars followed by split thickness skin graft (STSG) coverage.[5] Cutaneous flaps, Z-plasties, fasciocutaneous flaps, and musculocutaneous flaps may be required. Although the end goal is to reduce mammary volume, additional local tissue may need to be brought into the breast mound to improve contour before reduction mammaplasty. An inverted T incision with STSG between the breasts in the midline may be required to relax scar tissue over the breast mounds in the case of bilateral breast entrapment (**Fig. 1**). Some advocate for correction of NAC distortion at this time as well.

Delay Until Grafts Are Sufficiently Healed and Breasts Are Fully Developed

Grafts should be allowed to heal for at least 6 months and until the breasts are fully developed. Some investigators note that surgery is indicated when there is bulging of the breast tissue in an unburned area or when the scarred skin is obviously restricting breast growth.[6]

Be Conservative When Designing the Resection Pattern

The approach to reduction mammaplasty in burned patients is similar to that used in patients with symptomatic macromastia. As emphasized in Thai and colleagues,[4] moderately thick skin flaps (1.5–2.0 cm) and limited undermining will decrease the risk of flap necrosis. When designing the keyhole area of the Wise pattern, anticipate that the inherent inelastic nature of the skin grafts preclude wide transposition or advancement of such flaps (**Fig. 2**).

Consider Balancing Procedures at the Same Time

Although burned breasts can reach normal size and position, they differ from unburned breasts in their response to aging and development of ptosis. Thick scar contractures and the inelastic nature of the STSG serve as a sling that prevents the burned breast from becoming ptotic with aging. This asymmetry is most obvious in patients with only one burned breast; balancing procedures, such as mastopexy or reduction of the unburned breast, are recommended at the same time to restore

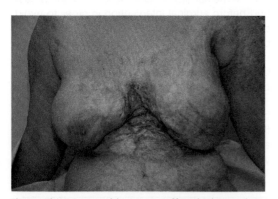

Fig. 1. This 21-year-old woman suffered a burn of the anterior chest wall in childhood with multiple subsequent debridements and skin grafting. She later underwent multiple scar contracture releases, including a midline inverted T incision with skin grafting over the sternum to improve breast contour and a laterally based fasciocutaneous flap to release and create the left breast inframammary fold.

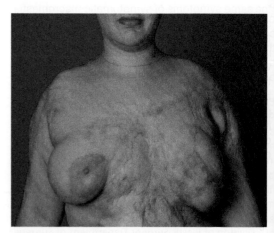

Fig. 2. This patient's full-thickness burn over the midline anterior chest both destroyed and distorted the breast parenchyma of both medial breasts. Any tissue mobilization medially should include thick skin flaps and conservation transposition.

symmetry.[4] Several investigators note that the excess skin generated by the mammaplasty can be used to release contractures or resurface unstable scarring in another burned area.[7]

As Payne and Malata[8] noted, the choice of surgical technique to correct postburn breast asymmetry and the associated macromastia is often complicated; the ideal technique should simultaneously address the skin contracture, nipple dystopia, and volume asymmetry.

TECHNICAL CONSIDERATIONS
Inferior Pedicle Mammaplasty

As El-Khatib[9] noted, the use of the inferior pedicle technique in burned breasts can solve many problems and the inferior pedicle dermal flap can be harvested from within the postburn scar. This technique reduces the size of large breasts, eliminates the scar tissue of the medial and lateral flaps, and brings the displaced NAC into a normal position.

Breast marking

Reduction mammaplasty in burned patients must be planned carefully. While patients are upright before the induction of anesthesia, the standard keyhole pattern is marked for the vertical dermal procedures as described by Strombeck[10] and McKissock.[11] As previously noted, when designing the keyhole area of the Wise pattern, anticipate that the inherent inelastic nature of the skin grafts precludes wide transposition or advancement of the skin flaps.

Take care to accommodate discrepancies between burned breasts or between a burned and unburned breast. Often the volume of specific poles or of the breasts overall are unequal. When compared with a contralateral unburned breast, the inframammary fold of the burned breast can be higher or even effaced secondary to scarring or contracture (see **Fig. 1**).

Excision and closure

As El-Khatib[9] noted, begin by releasing any burn contracture from the anterior chest wall and then marking the inferior dermal-parenchymal flap intraoperatively. All de-epithelization must be performed sharply because of the subdermal fibrosis of the burn scar. As mentioned previously, maintain 1.5- to 2.0-cm thickness of both medial and lateral flaps to preserve maximum blood supply to the overlying burnt skin. The NAC is transposed into the new position, and the procedure is completed in the standard fashion. Any secondary defects after release of the breast contracture can be grafted.

Superior Pedicle Mammaplasty

Relocation of the NAC of a burned breast to a more natural position often requires more flexibility than an inferior pedicle mammaplasty can provide. In those cases, a superomedial pedicle often can mobilize an inferiorly tethered NAC into a more anatomic relationship.[12]

Breast marking

A superior or superomedial pedicle combined with a LeJour-Lassus mastopexy technique can often provide the appropriate volume reduction and superior transposition of the NAC.[13] As with the inferior pedicle mammaplasty technique, skin flaps will likely be inelastic so 1.5-cm to 2.0-cm flap thickness should be maintained.

Excision and closure

As with the inferior pedicle mammaplasty, surgical release of any scar contractures should be performed first. This release allows for the superior pedicled transposition of the NAC. As Payne and Malata[8] noted, the Bostwick[14] modification of the LeJour vertical mammaplasty, including central wedge resection of excess breast tissue, minimal skin undermining, no hitching suture of the pedicle to the pectoral fascia, and minimal gathering of the vertical incision skin, can provide better results in the burned breast. The LeJour-Lassus lateral pillars, when approximated, recreate a stable conical breast mound where scarred skin and breast tissue have been resected inferiorly.

Recreation of the Inframammary Fold

The inframammary fold is often recreated with an inferiorly or laterally based fasciocutaneous flap (see **Fig. 1**). As Payne and Malata[8] noted, a modified Ryan procedure can also be used to recreate an amorphous inframammary fold even in the setting of a burned breast with macromastia.[15–27]

SUMMARY/DISCUSSION

Mammary hypertrophy can occur in the postburn breast, despite scarring and contractures. Patients with burned breasts exhibit the same symptoms of symptomatic macromastia as patients with unburned breasts do. The extent of the deformity, the location of the deformity, and the status of the surrounding soft tissue are all assessed before embarking on any surgical plan.

Although reduction in breast volume is the ultimate goal, improvement of breast contour through scar contracture release, through STSG and local tissue transfer, is undertaken first and allowed to fully heal as the breasts develop. During the reduction mammaplasty, regardless of technique, moderately thick skin flaps (1.5–2.0 cm) and limited undermining will decrease the risk of flap necrosis. The inherent inelastic nature of the skin grafts and scarred skin preclude wide transposition or advancement of skin flaps. Some investigators note that contralateral symmetry procedures are best performed simultaneously and that excised skin can be used for grafting a skin contracture elsewhere on the body.

Although many plastic surgeons are reluctant to operate on burned breasts for fear of devascularizing the skin graft or NAC, reduction mammaplasty in this group of patients is safe and carries minimal risk if key concepts are followed.

REFERENCES

1. Burns BF, McCauley RL, Murphy FL, et al. Reconstructive management of patients with greater than 80 percent TBSA burns. Burns 1993;19(5):429–33.

2. McCauley RL, Beraja V, Rutan RL, et al. Longitudinal assessment of breast development in adolescent female patients with burns involving the nipple-areolar complex. Plast Reconstr Surg 1989;83(4): 676–80.

3. McCauley RL, Killyon GW, Bowen K. Reconstruction of the burned breast and nipple-areolar complex. In: McCauley RL, editor. Functional and aesthetic reconstruction of burned patients. 1st edition. Boca Raton: CRC Press; 2005. p. 379–91.

4. Thai KN, Mertens D, Warden G, et al. Reduction mammaplasty in postburn breasts. Plast Reconstr Surg 1999;103(7):1882–6.

5. Neale HW, Smith GL, Gregory RO, et al. Breast reconstruction in the burned adolescent female (an 11-year, 157 patient experience). Plast Reconstr Surg 1982;70:718–24.

6. MacLennan SE, Wells MD, Neale HW. Reconstruction of the burned breast. Clin Plast Surg 2000;27: 113–9.

7. Shelley OP, Van Niekerk W, Cuccia G, et al. Dual benefit procedures: combining aesthetic surgery with burn reconstruction. Burns 2006;32:1022–7.

8. Payne CE, Malata CM. Correction of postburn breast asymmetry using the LeJour-type mammaplasty. Plast Reconstr Surg 2003;111(2):805–8.

9. El-Khatib H. Reliability of inferior pedicle reduction mammaplasty in burned oversized breasts. Plast Reconstr Surg 1999;103(3):869–73.

10. Strombeck JOP. Mammaplasty: report of a new technique based on the two pedicle procedure. Br J Plast Surg 1960;13:79.

11. McKissock PK. Reduction mammaplasty with a vertical dermal flap. Plast Reconstr Surg 1972;49:245.

12. Abulezz T. Mammoplasty in correcting scar-induced breast deformities. Ann Burns Fire Disasters 2009; 22(4):208–11.

13. LeJour M, Abboud M. Vertical mammaplasty without inframammary scar and with breast liposuction. Perspect Plast Surg 1990;4:67.

14. Bostwick J. Vertical mammaplasty: update and appraisal of late results. Plast Reconstr Surg 1999; 104:782 [discussion: 782–4].

15. Ryan JJ. A lower thoracic advancement flap in breast reconstruction after mastectomy. Plast Reconstr Surg 1982;70:153.

16. Armour AD, Billmire DA. Pediatric thermal injury: acute care and reconstruction update. Plast Reconstr Surg 2009;124(1):117e–27e.

17. Sadove AM, van Aalst JA. Congenital and acquired pediatric breast anomalies: a review of 20 years' experience. Plast Reconstr Surg 2005;115(4): 1039–50.

18. Pryor LS, Lehman JA, Workman MC. Disorders of the female breast in the pediatric age group. Plast Reconstr Surg 2009;124(1):50e–60e.

19. Ribas JMMR. Breast problems and diseases in puberty. Best Pract Res Clin Obstet Gynaecol 2010; 24:223–42.

20. Loss M, Infanger M, Kunzi W, et al. The burned female breast: a report on four cases. Burns 2002; 28:601–5.

21. Perez del Palomar A, Calvo B, Herrero J, et al. A finite element model to accurately predict real deformations of the breast. Med Eng Phys 2008; 30:1089–97.

22. Ozgur F, Gokalan I, Mavili E, et al. Reconstruction of postburn breast deformities. Burns 1992;18(6): 504–9.

23. Foley P, Jeeves A, Davey RB, et al. Breast burns are not benign: long-term outcomes of burns to the breast in pre-pubertal girls. Burns 2008;34:412–7.

24. Palao R, Gomez P, Huguet P. Burned breast reconstructive surgery with Integra dermal regenerative template. Br J Plast Surg 2003;56:252–9.

25. Hsiao YC, Yang JY, Chuang SS, et al. Are augmentation mammaplasty and reconstruction of the burned breast collateral lines? Experience in performing simultaneous reconstructive and aesthetic surgery. Burns 2009;35:130–6.

26. Bayram Y, Sahin C, Sever C, et al. Custom-made approach to a patient with post-burn breast deformity. Indian J Plast Surg 2014;47(1):127–31.

27. Yesilada AK, Sevim KZ, Sirvan SS, et al. Our surgical approach to treatment of congenital, developmental, and acquired breast asymmetries: a review of 30 cases. Aesthetic Plast Surg 2013;37(1):77–87.

Avoiding Complications in Gigantomastia

Russell E. Kling, MD, William D. Tobler Jr, MD, Jeffrey A. Gusenoff, MD, J. Peter Rubin, MD*

KEYWORDS

- Gigantomastia • Complications • Surgical breast reduction

KEY POINTS

- Gigantomastia represents extreme hypertrophy of the female breast.
- Although there is no universally accepted definition, the amount of tissue resected during reduction mammaplasty is the most widely used description, with threshold ranges reported between 1000 g and 2000 g per breast.
- Gigantomastia is a complicated problem that presents unique challenges. Understanding the cause of the disease and the necessary preoperative workup will minimize complications from the operation.
- There are multiple surgical approaches for correcting gigantomastia. Although there is not one best approach, many standard approaches can be adapted with an understanding of how to maintain blood supply to the nipple/areolar complex.
- As a general guideline, a pedicle width (when pedicles are used) of at least 8 cm should be maintained with a pedicle length no more than twice that of the width.

INTRODUCTION

Gigantomastia is a disabling condition for patients and presents unique challenges to the plastic surgeon. Excessive breast tissue is associated with pain in the back, neck, and shoulders. These patients often have intertrigo and can have derangements in body image perception, quality of life, and physical functioning.[1] To this day, the definition of this condition remains unsettled. There are multiple causes, the most common of which is idiopathic.[2,3] Presentation can occur throughout different phases of life, and treatment often begins with nonoperative measures; however, the most effective way to relieve symptoms is surgical breast reduction.[4,5] Because of the large amount of tissue removed, surgeons can encounter different intraoperative and postoperative complications. By understanding this disease process and these complications, surgeons can attempt to minimize their occurrences. The authors present an overview of the cause, preoperative evaluation, techniques, and outcomes. Additionally, they present outcomes data from their center on 40 patients.

DEFINITION

The amount of tissue resected during a reduction mammaplasty is often used as a marker and definition for gigantomastia. However, there is wide disagreement about how much excised tissue weight constitutes gigantomastia, with ranges between 1000 g per breast and as high as 2000 g per breast reported in the literature.[6–9] Definitions focusing on body mass index (BMI), brassiere size, and breast size also exist. In an attempt to standardize the categorization of gigantomastia, Dancey and colleagues[3] proposed a new classification system based on cause, age, BMI, and pregnancy status (**Table 1**).

Department of Plastic Surgery, University of Pittsburgh, Pittsburgh, PA 15260, USA
* Corresponding author.
E-mail address: rubipj@UPMC.EDU

Clin Plastic Surg 43 (2016) 429–439
http://dx.doi.org/10.1016/j.cps.2015.12.006

Table 1
Dancey classification of gigantomastia

Group	Characteristics
1a	Idiopathic, spontaneous condition of excessive breast growth in patients with a BMI >30
1b	Idiopathic, spontaneous condition of excessive breast growth in patients with a BMI <30
2a	Excessive breast growth related to an imbalance of endogenous hormone production occurring during puberty
2b	Excessive breast growth related to an imbalance of endogenous hormone production occurring during pregnancy
3	Excessive breast growth induced by a pharmacologic agent

Another possibly more objective definition from Dafydd and colleagues[10] proposes using excessive breast tissue that contributes 3% or more to patients' total body weight. For the purposes of the data presented from the authors' hospital in this article, they chose 1500 g per breast as their benchmark resection weight and definition of gigantomastia.

CAUSES

There are several different causes for gigantomastia. The most common cause is idiopathic[2,3] (**Box 1**). This condition can also be seen in

Box 1
Etiology of gigantomastia

Idiopathic

Pregnancy induced

Puberty induced

Pharmacologic

   Penicillamine

   Neothetazone

   Cyclosporine

   Estrogen

   Bucillamine

Autoimmune

   Chronic arthritis

   Hashimoto thyroiditis

   Myasthenia gravis

   Psoriasis

association with pregnancy and puberty. Pregnancy-induced gigantomastia occurs with an incidence of approximately 1 in 65,000 pregnancies. Characteristic features of puberty- and pregnancy-induced gigantomastia include glandular hyperplasia, hyperplasia of the stromal elements, and fibrosis.[4] There are also reports of gigantomastia developing as a result of medication side effects and autoimmune disease.[2,3,11]

ANATOMY

Gross[12] (**Fig. 1**)

- There are certain key features that are present in patients with macromastia and gigantomastia. These features include severe ptosis, increased sternal notch to nipple distance, increased nipple to inframammary fold (IMF) distance, increased areolar size, and a broadened base. Understanding the vascular supply to the nipple-areola complex (NAC) is imperative for a safe and effective operation. The NAC is supplied by the internal mammary artery, lateral thoracic artery at the level of the fourth intercostal artery, and the anterior intercostal artery at the level of the midfourth and fifth intercostal spaces.

Histology[13]

- There are also histologic changes that are present in gigantomastia, which can differ with the varying causes. Idiopathic gigantomastia demonstrates predominantly fibroglandular tissue, lymphocytic infiltration, and venostasis. The hormonal subtype shows stromal, ductal, and glandular hyperplasia with dilatation. In addition, the histology shows collagenous fibrosis, cellular myxoid hyperplasia, ductal proliferation with cystic degeneration, edema, lymphatic dilatation, and fibroadenomas with increased estrogen and progesterone. Interestingly, drug-induced gigantomastia does not show any significant histologic changes.[3]

EVALUATION

All women presenting with severe breast hypertrophy require a *complete* history and physical examination. A thorough weight history should be obtained, including weight loss surgery, lowest/highest/current weight, and how breast size has changed with weight. In addition, history of any breast abnormalities, including masses and/or prior surgeries, should be obtained.[1,14] Breastfeeding history should be discussed as well as any future plans for breastfeeding, which could be compromised by surgical intervention. Family

A

B

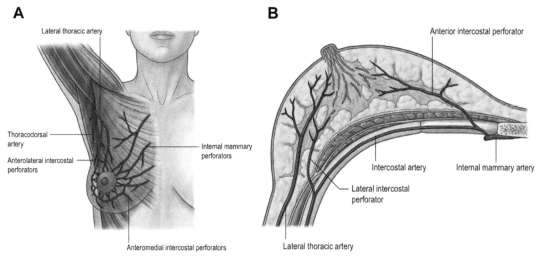

Fig. 1. (*A*) Shows the arterial supply to the breast in an anterior view, and (*B*) shows the blood supply in a cross sectional view. (*From* de la Torre J, Davis MR. Anatomy for plastic surgery of the breast. In: Neligan PC, editor. Plastic surgery, vol. 5. Breast, Chapter 1. 3rd edition. Philadelphia: Elsevier, Saunders; 2013. p. 7; with permission.)

history of cancer, including breast, ovarian, or co-lon, should be discussed.

- The physical examination begins with a general inspection of patients and the topography of the breasts, noting any asymmetries, position of the NAC, presence of any chest wall rolls, scars, and quality of skin. A complete breast examination should be performed evaluating any masses, the position and mobility of the IMF, and nipple sensation. Finally anatomic measurements should be performed, which include suprasternal notch to nipple, midclavicle to nipple, nipple to IMF, breast base, and NAC size.

Treatment Options

Conservative management
- Properly fitted brassiere
- Physical therapy
- Weight reduction

Medical management
- Medical management of gigantomastia is based on a limited number of case reports and is grouped in the literature based on cause. Medical management and noninterventional methods often fail and, thus, surgery is required.
  - Pregnancy induced
    - Bromocriptine, the most commonly used medication for this disease, is a dopamine agonist, which centrally inhibits the release of prolactin and produces a

temporary involution of breast tissue during pregnancy. Despite this therapy, most women still require surgical correction after treatment. Other agents that have been tried with pregnancy-induced gigantomastia include androgens, estrogens, progestins, 2 bromine-alpha ergocryptine, prednisone, dexamethasone, hydrochlorothiazide, and furosemide with either marginal or no effects seen.
- Idiopathic and puberty induced
  - Tamoxifen, an estrogen receptor antagonist, has been shown to cause regression of breast tissue. Other agents that have been tried include medroxyprogesterone and dydrogesterone.[3]

Preoperative Counseling

Overview
- A preoperative patient-surgeon counseling session *is of the utmost importance.* Asymmetry should be discussed with patients. Although each breast may appear similar to patients preoperatively, even small differences in size postoperatively may be observed by patients. The goals of the procedure need to be highlighted during preoperative counseling, and the potential need for free nipple grafting must be discussed.

Goals of reduction mammaplasty in gigantomastia
- Breast volume reduction sufficient to eliminate symptoms

- Elevating the NAC
- Tightening the skin envelope
- Correcting severe asymmetry
- Reshaping the breast mound[1,15]

Other Preoperative Considerations

- It may be necessary to involve an endocrine specialist, especially in pregnant or pubescent-aged girls. Prior algorithms have been established specifically for the gestational patient population.[4] Of note, reduction mammaplasty for these patients does *not* reduce the rate of recurrence in subsequent pregnancies. The likelihood of future pregnancy is a key determinant of the type of procedure offered (**Fig. 2**).[4]

Surgical Management

Overview

- Surgical management is the most effective treatment of gigantomastia. Although there are several different surgical options, the literature to date only reports small series specific to this patient population and optimal techniques. In cases requiring more than 1000 g per breast resected, surgeons should consider free nipple grafting, although some have argued for a more liberal cutoff at 2000 g per breast. The cutoff should depend on both operator experience and comfort level with the procedure. Additional consideration should be given to high-risk patients. Regardless of surgeon preference, a thorough patient discussion is recommended to discuss the risks, benefits, and alternatives of each proposed procedure. There are many different techniques described, including inferior, superomedial, medial, and bipedicled flaps; the most pertinent topics to address severe breast hypertrophy are described later (**Figs. 3** and **4**).

Selecting a surgical technique

- Preoperative markings are an important determinant of symmetry and shape and contribute greatly to surgical planning.

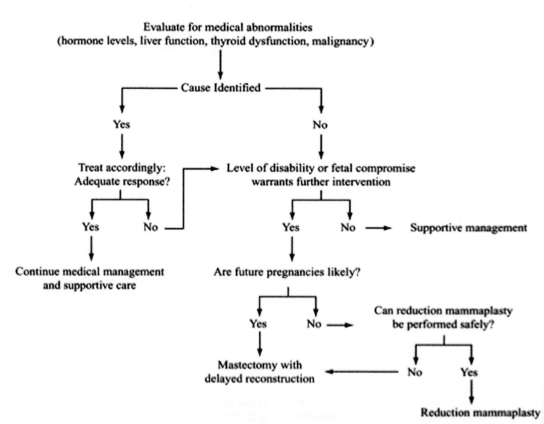

Fig. 2. Treatment algorithm for gestational gigantomastia. (*From* Swelstad MR, Swelstad BB, Rao VK, et al. Management of gestational gigantomastia. Plast Reconstr Surg 2006;118(4):845; with permission.)

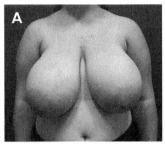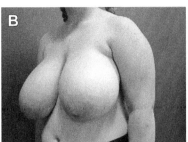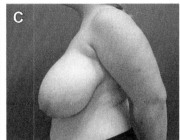

Fig. 3. Preoperative photographs demonstrating anteroposterior (*A*), oblique (*B*), and lateral (*C*) views of an 18-year-old patient with gigantomastia.

Superiorly based pedicles work best with short sternal notch to nipple distances, whereas inferiorly based pedicles tend to work best with short IMF to nipple distances. Typically, for vertical scar reduction, mammaplasty sternal notch to nipple distance should be less than 38 cm. Likewise, when the IMF to nipple distance is more than 22 cm, the inferior pedicle is not recommended. There is a risk of poor blood supply to the NAC as well as a risk of kinking of the pedicle, which could compromise the viability of the NAC. Alternatively, if the aforementioned techniques will still compromise blood flow, then a safe option is to perform a free nipple graft.[16] In order to avoid complications and for optimal results, the choice of surgical technique should be based on breast morphology.

- In patients with gigantomastia, the weight of the breast can distort the IMF inferiorly. Therefore, careful assessment of each IMF is critical. Additionally, in extremely large breasts, the parenchyma is displaced laterally, which requires medial displacement before marking of the meridian in order for most of the breast mound to be under the central meridian.[17]

Inferior pedicle reduction mammaplasty
- Pedicle-based breast reduction, now the standard of care for breast hypertrophy, has also shown good outcomes in uniquely challenging gigantomastia patients.[18–20] Lacerna and colleagues[9] published their experience since 1984 of 219 inferior pedicle reduction mammaplasties for gigantomastia without a single case requiring nipple grafting. Postoperatively, the most frequent complication they noted was widening of the inferior portion of the inverted T incision, occurring 7% to 20% of the time.[9,21–23] Although they were able to demonstrate success without free nipple grafting, a surgeon must always be prepared to convert to a free nipple graft if needed. The most important factor is the clinical determination of adequate blood flow to the NAC. There is not a defined critical pedicle length set as a cutoff for free nipple grafting, so the surgeon must make a decision intraoperatively about the viability of the NAC. If there are any signs of impending necrosis, such as decreased capillary refill or mottling of tissues, then free nipple grafting can and should be performed as a safe alternative.

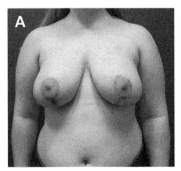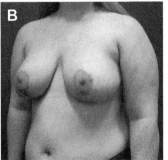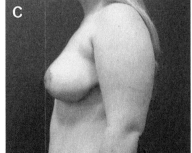

Fig. 4. Postoperative photographs demonstrating anteroposterior (*A*), oblique (*B*), and lateral (*C*) views 5.5 months after Wise pattern reduction mammaplasty with an inferior pedicle. Excised tissue weights were 1420 g on the left and 1543 g on the right. The patient had a superficial dehiscence along the vertical incision of the right breast. This dehiscence healed by secondary intention with local wound care.

- A variation of the inverted T reduction mammaplasty that has also shown success in the gigantomastia patient is the no vertical scar reduction.[24–26] This technique transposes the NAC via an IMF and periareolar incision without making a vertical incision.[25,26] In an article by Degeorge and colleagues,[17] most of the largest breasts were reduced in this manner. They achieved a "mature breast shape"[17] with few complications compared with the Wise pattern. However, they did note "less central projection" and "lack of narrowing at the base of the breast."[17]
- The short scar periareolar inferior pedicle reduction (SPAIR) technique developed by Hammond is another variation of the inferior pedicle technique. This technique combines the safety of the inferior pedicle with reduced IMF scarring and long-term rates of bottoming out. SPAIR is versatile and in experienced hands can be applied to breast reductions involving more then 1000 g per breast.[27]
- Keys to the dissection
  ○ Dissect the superior flap to the clavicle level for sufficient pedicle coverage.
  ○ Flaps should remain at least 2 cm thick.
  ○ Maintain a wide pedicle at least 8 cm to avoid nipple necrosis.
  ○ Avoid thinning the pedicle during dissection by flaring out at the base.
  ○ Maintain medial fullness by avoiding over-resection.

Superomedial reduction mammaplasty
- An advantage to the superomedial approach is that it maintains the dominant medially based internal mammary perforators.[28] Also there is improved long-term projection because the inferior tissue, which contributes to bottoming out, is resected. Furthermore, the procedure is associated with a reduced rate of skin necrosis because skin flap undermining is usually not required for closure. The superior aspect of the superomedial pedicle creates a wider pedicle versus the medial pedicle, which is advisable in this high-risk group. However, widening the pedicle width limits the arc of rotation to about 90°.[8,29,30] Landau and Hudson[31] noted a minor areola slough rate of 6.5%, but most importantly 100% had viable nipples postoperatively. A particularly high T-junction breakdown rate of 18% was also observed.[31]
- Another option is to perform a superomedial reduction using only a vertical scar. Lugo and colleagues[32] reported on their 12-year

experience with 200 cases of gigantomastia. The cohort had an average partial NAC necrosis rate of 10.5%, and only 2% lost nipple sensation.
- Keys to the dissection
  ○ Preserve medial attachments to the chest wall avoiding vascular supply from internal mammary artery and vein.
  ○ Maintain a wide pedicle and flare out at the base.
  ○ Avoid twisting the pedicle and obstructing the blood supply.
  ○ Use a back cut when needed to position the pedicle.

Reduction with free nipple grafts
- Reduction mammaplasty with free nipple grafting has traditionally been the gold standard treatment of severe breast hypertrophy; however, it is now considered, by most, to be a salvage or last-resort procedure.[9,33,34] Over time the technique has been refined, and today free nipple grafting can be combined with pedicle-based reduction mammaplasty (**Fig. 5**).
- Although free nipple grafting will diminish the risk of NAC loss, it is associated with its own complications, specifically loss of NAC sensation.[35–39] Other issues include lack of nipple projection, ptosis, nipple hypopigmentation, and loss of lactation. It is important to review all of these outcome possibilities with patients before embarking on this procedure. Free nipple grafting should not be performed in women of childbearing age who plan to breastfeed or in women who want to preserve nipple sensation and erection.
- Keys to the dissection
  ○ Mark the Wise pattern preoperatively, paying attention to nipple position and avoiding placement too high on the breast. Nipple position may need to be set lower than a traditional breast reduction.
  ○ The inverted V shape may need to be wider than in standard reductions in order to avoid incorporating the native areola into the vertical scar. However, small peripheral areola inclusion can be tolerated.
  ○ Resect the nipple as a full-thickness graft, and defat as needed.
  ○ Apply a tie-over bolster to the free nipple graft and remove 1 week postoperatively.

Complications

The authors reviewed their own institution's experience (n = 40) with gigantomastia reduction mammaplasty. Inclusion criteria included resections

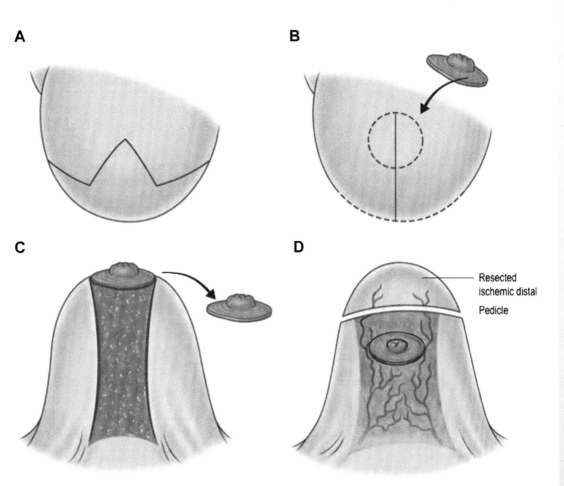

Fig. 5. Removing the NAC from its present position and replacing it on more proximally on the breast pedicle as a full thickness skin graft (*A, B*). The nipple graft can also be placed on a de-epithelialized area of the breast skin flaps (*C, D*). (*Reprinted from* Shestak K. Revision surgery following breast reduction and mastopexy. In: Neligan PC, editor. Plastic Surgery, vol. 5. Breast, Chapter 9. 3rd edition. Philadelphia: Elsevier, Saunders; 2013. p. 248; with permission.)

greater than 1500 g in at least one breast. Oncoplastic breast reductions were not excluded. Refer to **Table 2** for the authors' institution's complications and outcomes. The authors' results are consistent with other studies examining complications after gigantomastia (**Tables 3** and **4**). The authors also performed an analysis of variance to examine preferred technique versus complications, which resulted in a *P* value of .100 at a 0.05 significance level. The authors then conducted a Pearson correlation for BMI versus complication, which resulted in $r^2 = 0.146$, $P = .381$. These analyses, therefore, demonstrate that technique and BMI are *not* significantly correlated with complication rates.

Nipple-Areola Complex Necrosis

Procedure selection can help reduce the risk of NAC necrosis. An important decision is whether to perform a free nipple graft. General guidelines include using a sternal notch to nipple distance greater than 40 cm, IMF to nipple distance greater than 20 cm, age greater than 65 years, patient comorbidities, and surgeon preference as thresholds for considering free nipple grafting. Although the authors do not advocate for a particular pedicle, maximizing pedicle width is a good practice. Postoperative NAC necrosis, when it occurs, is most often partial thickness. This complication can often be treated with local wound care alone, and it usually heals without issue. When NAC necrosis becomes full thickness, sharp debridement is needed and may ultimately require NAC reconstruction.

Hematoma

Hematoma formation following large-volume breast reduction remains a significant problem. A combination of good surgical technique and

Table 2
Retrospective analysis of outcomes in gigantomastia reduction mammaplasty at the University of Pittsburgh from 2004 to 2015: complications in 40 patient series

Average weight resected per breast (g)	1886 (SD 673; range 1518–4309)
Average age (y)	41.2 (SD 15; range 17–71)
Free nipple graft	28% *1 case of a converted free nipple graft*
Wound dehiscence	25% *90% managed with conservative wound care*
Cellulitis (requiring oral antibiotics)	10%
Elective scar revision	5%
Reoperation, nonelective	5%
NAC partial-thickness necrosis	7.5% *1 case was a free nipple graft*
Hematoma requiring evacuation	2.5%
Seroma (requiring aspiration)	2.5%
NAC full-thickness necrosis	2.5%

perioperative management can minimize the risk of hematoma formation. This combination includes controlling perioperative blood pressure, postoperative compression dressings, holding antiplatelet agents perioperatively, and smoking cessation. Postoperative pain and nausea should be controlled to avoid abrupt elevations in blood pressure. To this end, the authors advocate for incisional local anesthesia and antiemetics as needed. Although there is strong level I and II evidence against prophylactic subcutaneous drains, this specific patient population has not been evaluated in a particular study.[40–44]

Seroma

Seroma formation can cause patient discomfort and delay return to normal life. Seroma formation can be managed on an outpatient basis with serial needle aspiration with most resolving clinically within 1 month.

Wound Dehiscence

Wound dehiscence is the most frequent complication following breast reduction surgery occurring most commonly at the T-point junction. The most cited cause includes infection and high tension on the wound edges. Other risk factors include tobacco use, lengthy operative times, obesity, and large resection volumes. Local wound management and healing by secondary intention is appropriate for partial dehiscence. Management options include topical antibiotic preparations, moist dressings, silver-hydrofiber dressings, and negative-pressure therapy. For cases with significant dehiscence, operative intervention may be needed.

Wound Infection

Wound infection following reduction mammaplasty remains a persistent problem for both the surgeon and patients alike. There is strong level I evidence to support the use of preoperative antibiotics. Preoperative antibiotics can reduce infection rates by 75%. The use of antibiotics postoperatively is uncertain. No high-level evidence supports the use of topical antibiotics in breast operations.[45]

Nipple-Areola Complex Sensation Disturbances

NAC sensation disturbances can be quite concerning to patients. Patients undergoing inferior pedicle reductions typically realize restoration of normal preoperative sensation within 6 to 12 months. The surgical technique and not the amount of breast tissue resected influences postoperative NAC sensation. The technique most associated with NAC sensation disturbances is the superior pedicle technique.[46] The lateral cutaneous nerves, the dominant nerves supplying the NAC, are resected with the base of the breast. Patients are keenly aware of nipple disturbances; accordingly a discussion of surgical technique and its implications on sensation should be had with patients.

SUMMARY

Gigantomastia is a debilitating condition both physically and emotionally. Historically, the most dependable procedure for this condition was free nipple grafting. However, newer case series have shown that nipple transposition in conjunction with pedicle-based reductions can achieve equivalent to better results. The most frequent complications following gigantomastia reductions are wound healing issues that are usually self-limited and heal well with local wound care. Specific guidelines for considering preoperative free nipple grafting are loosely defined but this option should

Table 3
Examining outcomes in gigantomastia reduction mammaplasty in the literature: complication rates in the published literature

Study	Technique	Cohort Size	Resection Size (g)	Complication Rates
Lacerna et al	Inferior pedicle with inverted T scar	15	Minimum of 2000 g/breast	1 case of partial-thickness NAC necrosis, 0 cases of full-thickness NAC necrosis
Mojallal et al	Posterosuperior pedicle with inverted T scar	50	Average of 1231 g/breast	1 case (2%) of partial-thickness NAC necrosis, 1 case of infection requiring I&D, 6 cases (12%) of delayed wound healing T incision
Heine et al	Superior-based pedicle with a short vertical scar	25	Minimum of 1000 g/breast	5 (20%) had minor complications, including scar dehiscence, hypertrophic scars, and local healing problems; 3 (12%) had major complications, including wound infection, local fat necrosis, and a late seroma
Nahabedian et al	Medial pedicle with inverted T scar	23	Average of 1604 g/breast	1 case converted to a free nipple graft, 100% of nipples viable postoperatively, 98% of cases maintained NAC sensation, 1 case of requiring contour revision
Lugo et al	Superomedial pedicle with inverted T scar	200	Average of 1280 g/breast	21 (10.5%) cases of partial necrosis of NAC; 98% normal NAC sensation postoperatively
Costa et al	Superior medial pedicle with inverted T scar	90	Average of 1400 g/breast	1 case of hematoma (1%), 1 case of seroma (1%), 0 cases of infection, 0 cases of full-thickness NAC necrosis, 3 cases of dehiscence (3%)
Azzam et al	Vertical scar mammaplasty using the modified Lejour technique	53	Minimum of 1000 g/breast	0 cases of hematoma, 3 cases of seroma, 2 cases of partial NAC necrosis, 1 case of total NAC necrosis, 10 cases of dehiscence, 1 case of infection, 12 cases requiring scar revision, 1 cases requiring volume revision
Landau et al	Superomedial pedicle with inverted T scar	61	Average of 1360 g/breast	8 cases of partial areola necrosis (6.5%), 22 cases of T-junction breakdown (18%), 0 cases of full-thickness NAC necrosis

Table 4
Examining outcomes in nongigantomastia reduction mammaplasty in the literature: complication rates in the published literature

Study	Cohort Size	Average Weight Resected (g)	Complication Rates
Manhan et al	1148	900	Wounds 14.9%, scars 14.5%, surgical scar 6.7% revision, 7.3% infection, 1.2% seroma
Lewin et al	512	468	Delayed wound healing 10.5%, partial-thickness NAC necrosis 11.5%, full-thickness NAC necrosis 0.6%, grade 2 or higher infection 11%, reoperation 1.4%

always be considered. Surgeon experience and patient goals need to also be considered when planning a gigantomastia reduction. The surgeon should have a diverse and thorough understanding of all the surgical techniques for gigantomastia so that operative planning can be based on each patients particular breast morphology and not just on the comfort level of the surgeon.

REFERENCES

1. Kalliainen LK, ASPS Health Policy Committee. ASPS clinical practice guideline summary on reduction mammaplasty. Plast Reconstr Surg 2012;130(4): 785–9.

2. Cho MJ, Yang JH, Choi HG, et al. An idiopathic gigantomastia. Ann Surg Treat Res 2015;88(3):166–9.

3. Dancey A, Khan M, Dawson J, et al. Gigantomastia–a classification and review of the literature. J Plast Reconstr Aesthet Surg 2008;61(5):493–502.

4. Swelstad MR, Swelstad BB, Rao VK, et al. Management of gestational gigantomastia. Plast Reconstr Surg 2006;118(4):840–8.

5. Bloom SA, Nahabedian MY. Gestational macromastia: a medical and surgical challenge. Breast J 2008; 14(5):492–5.

6. Azzam C, De Mey A. Vertical scar mammaplasty in gigantomastia: retrospective study of 115 patients treated using the modified Lejour technique. Aesthetic Plast Surg 2007;31(3):294–8.

7. Ozçelik D, Unveren T, Toplu G, et al. Vertical mammaplasty for gigantomastia. Aesthetic Plast Surg 2009;33(2):246–9.

8. Costa MP, Ching AW, Ferreira MC. Thin superior medial pedicle reduction mammaplasty for severe mammary hypertrophy. Aesthetic Plast Surg 2008; 32(4):645–52.

9. Lacerna M, Spears J, Mitra A, et al. Avoiding free nipple grafts during reduction mammaplasty in patients with gigantomastia. Ann Plast Surg 2005; 55(1):21–4.

10. Dafydd H, Roehl KR, Phillips LG, et al. Redefining gigantomastia. J Plast Reconstr Aesthet Surg 2011;64(2):160–3.

11. Troccola A, Maruccia M, Dessy LA, et al. Cortisone-induced gigantomastia during chemotherapy. G Chir 2011;32(5):266–9.

12. de la Torre J, Davis MR. Anatomy for plastic surgery of the breast. In: Neligan PC, editor. Plastic surgery, vol. 5. Breast, Chapter 1. 3rd edition. Philadelphia: Elsevier, Saunders; 2013. p. 1–13.

13. Lafreniere R, Temple W, Ketcham A. Gestational macromastia. Am J Surg 1984;148(3):413–8.

14. Toy J, Rubin JP. Contouring of the arms, breast, upper trunk, and male chest in the massive weight loss patient. In: Neligan PC, editor. Plastic surgery, vol. 5. Breast, Chapter 24. 3rd edition. Philadelphia: Elsevier, Saunders; 2013. p. 557–82.

15. Hammond DC, Loffredo M. Breast reduction. Plast Reconstr Surg 2012;129(5):829e–39e.

16. Fisher J, Higdon K. Reduction mammoplasty. In: Neligan P, editor. Plastic surgery, vol. 5. Breast, Chapter 8. 3rd edition. Philadelphia: Elsevier, Saunders; 2013. p. 152–64.

17. Degeorge BR Jr, Colen DL, Mericli AF, et al. Reduction mammoplasty operative techniques for improved outcomes in the treatment of gigantomastia. Eplasty 2013;13:e54.

18. Georgiade GS, Riefkohl RE, Georgiade NG. The inferior dermal-pyramidal type breast reduction: long-term evaluation. Ann Plast Surg 1989;23(3):203–11.

19. Ribeiro L. A new technique for reduction mammaplasty. Plast Reconstr Surg 1975;55(3):330–4.

20. Chang P, Shaaban AF, Canady JW, et al. Reduction mammaplasty: the results of avoiding nipple-areolar amputation in cases of extreme hypertrophy. Ann Plast Surg 1996;37(6):585–91.

21. Rohrich RJ, Gosman AA, Brown SA, et al. Current preferences for breast reduction techniques: a survey of board-certified plastic surgeons 2002. Plast Reconstr Surg 2004;114(7):1724–33 [discussion: 1734–6].

22. Heine N, Eisenmann-Klein M, Prantl L. Gigantomasty: treatment with a short vertical scar. Aesthetic Plast Surg 2008;32(1):41–7.

23. Amini P, Stasch T, Theodorou P, et al. Vertical reduction mammaplasty combined with a

superomedial pedicle in gigantomastia. Ann Plast Surg 2010;64:3–10.

24. Liu TS, Crisera CA, Festekjian JH, et al. Staged wise-pattern skin excision for reconstruction of the large and ptotic breast. Plast Reconstr Surg 2010;126: 1831–9.

25. Passot R. La correction esthetique du prolapsus mammaire par le procede de la transposition du mamelon. Presse Med 1925;33:317.

26. Lalonde DH, Lalonde J, French R. The no vertical scar breast reduction: a minor variation that allows to remove vertical scar portion of the inferior pedicle wise pattern T scar. Aesthetic Plast Surg 2003;27(5): 335–44.

27. Hammond DC. Short scar periareolar inferior pedicle reduction (SPAIR) mammaplasty. Plast Reconstr Surg 1999;103(3):890–901 [discussion: 902].

28. Palmer JH, Taylor GI. The vascular territories of the anterior chest wall. Br J Plast Surg 1986;39:287.

29. Finger RE, Vasquez B, Drew GS, et al. Superomedial pedicle technique of reduction mammaplasty. Plast Reconstr Surg 1989;83:471.

30. Lejour M. Vertical mammaplasty and liposuction of the breast. Plast Reconstr Surg 1994;94(1):100–14.

31. Landau AG, Hudson DA. Choosing the superomedial pedicle for reduction mammaplasty in gigantomastia. Plast Reconstr Surg 2008;121(3):735–9.

32. Lugo LM, Prada M, Kohanzadeh S, et al. Surgical outcomes of gigantomastia breast reduction superomedial pedicle technique: a 12-year retrospective study. Ann Plast Surg 2013;70(5):533–7.

33. McGregor JC, Hafeez A. Is there still a place for free nipple areolar grafting in breast reduction surgery? A review of cases over a three year period. J Plast Reconstr Aesthet Surg 2006;59:213–8 [discussion: 219–20].

34. Thorek M. Possibilities in the recognition of the human form. N Y Med J 1922;116:572.

35. Basaran K, Saydam FA, Ersin I, et al. The free-nipple breast-reduction technique performed with transfer of the nipple-areola complex over the superior or superomedial pedicles. Aesthetic Plast Surg 2014; 38(4):718–26.

36. Hawtof DB, Levine M, Kapetansky DI, et al. Complications of reduction mammaplasty: comparison of nipple-areolar graft and pedicle. Ann Plast Surg 1989;23(1):3–10.

37. Koger KE, Sunde D, Press BHJ, et al. Reduction mammaplasty for gigantomastia using inferior based pedicle and free nipple transplantation. Ann Plast Surg 1994;33:561.

38. Townsend PL. Nipple sensation following breast reduction and free nipple transplantation. Br J Plast Surg 1974;27:308–10.

39. Güven E, Aydin H, Başaran K, et al. Reduction mammaplasty using bipedicled dermoglandular flaps and free-nipple transplantation. Aesthetic Plast Surg 2010;34(6):738–44.

40. Hussien M, Lee S, Malyon A, et al. The impact of intraoperative hypotension on the development of wound haematoma after breast reduction. Br J Plast Surg 2001 Sep;54(6):517–22.

41. Kop EC, Spauwen PH, Kouwenberg PP, et al. Influence of controlled hypotension versus normotension on amount of blood loss during breast reduction. J Plast Reconstr Aesthet Surg 2009;62(2):200–5.

42. Kerrigan CL, Slezak SS. Evidence-based medicine: reduction mammaplasty. Plast Reconstr Surg 2013; 132(6):1670–83.

43. Collis N, McGuiness CM, Batchelor AG. Drainage in breast reduction surgery: a prospective randomised intra-patient trial. Br J Plast Surg 2005;58:286–9.

44. Corion LU, Smeulders MJ, van Zuijlen PP, et al. Draining after breast reduction: a randomised controlled inter-patient study. J Plast Reconstr Aesthet Surg 2009;62:865–8.

45. Shortt R, Cooper MJ, Farrokhyar F, et al. Meta-analysis of antibiotic prophylaxis in breast reduction surgery. Plast Surg (Oakv) 2014;22(2):91–4.

46. Schlenz I, Rigel S, Schemper M, et al. Alteration of nipple and areola sensitivity by reduction mammaplasty: a prospective comparison of five techniques. Plast Reconstr Surg 2005;115(3):743–51 [discussion: 752–4].

Medicolegal Issues in Breast Reduction

Neal R. Reisman, MD, JD

KEYWORDS

- Breast reduction risks • Consent • Malpractice

KEY POINTS

- Areas of general risk are discussed with patients before surgery.
- Procedure-specific risks inherent in each technique are a key part of informed consent.
- Issues related to insurance coverage must be settled preoperatively to decrease litigation risk.
- Protection of patient information has become a key part of the overall treatment process and this information must be protected.

Breast reduction surgery, a common procedure in plastic surgery has enjoyed high satisfaction ratings well into the mid-90% level. In recent years, however, breast reduction has risen to the second highest procedure associated with breast litigation. What has changed? It is unknown whether patient expectations have evolved beyond appropriate, if practices misrepresent the risks and concerns of this procedure, or if a general lack of patient accountability exists. Regardless of the reason, it behooves plastic surgeons to understand the increased risk of breast reduction and incorporate an appropriate amount of time and discussion to address concerns. First, this article is separated into areas of general risk, which include general scarring, infection, and anesthesia, to name some. Second, specific risks associated with scarring, loss of nipple areola, size, asymmetry, and laxity along with many patient misconceptions about the level the breast remain. Third, there are specific issues with insurance coverage that pose significant risks to patients at the practice. Last, in the digital age, there must be a discussion of protecting patient information, especially photographs, and other patient identified drawings and information used in the process known as informed consent.

GENERAL RISKS

General risks can be found in most informed consent documents and it is suggested that the included items be discussed and understood so that patients have an understanding of general risks with any surgery and anesthetic and of the preparation, preoperative, intraoperative, and postoperative requirements and instructions.

SPECIFIC RISKS

There are many specific risks attributable to breast reduction surgery. There are however specific risks associated with this procedure attributable to the many different techniques used that should be understood. I recall a lawsuit many years ago that I reviewed of a surgeon who showed photographs of bad thickened wide scars. The patient, however, had scars that were worse than the worst depiction shown to her. Surgeons must be careful to not represent the level of scarring or how bad scars may become or how good they might be over time. Every patient is different and it is important to not create a warrantee that will be discussed later about the end result. Smoking has been well shown to affect healing and can have devastating effects on breast reduction.

The author has no financial or commercial conflicts of interest.

Plastic Surgery, Baylor-St. Luke's Hospital, Baylor College of Medicine, Houston, TX, USA

E-mail address: drreisman@hotmail.com

Clin Plastic Surg 43 (2016) 441–444

http://dx.doi.org/10.1016/j.cps.2015.12.013

Generally it is recommended to stop any form of nicotine usage whether by nicotine patches or other nicotine related uses devices or a tobacco 3 to 4 weeks before the surgery date. I understand smoking is an addiction and some patients are dishonest or embarrassed to acknowledge they have not stopped; a urine cotinine test can detect nicotine usage up to a month prior. It is important that patients acknowledge they smoke and are aware of the effects of nicotine on potential loss of nipple areola and poor scars. Another issue arises when a practice becomes aware of a patient's continued use of tobacco. The warnings alone are not a protection to the practice if blood supply is affected. The practice may have a duty to cancel surgery and consider alternative means to protect and assist patients' results. I am aware of many instances where the surgery time is blocked and at the morning of surgery it becomes evident a patient has continued to smoke. Having the patient acknowledge the dangers is an advantage but the practice knowingly continuing to proceed with surgery may remove that help completely.[1]

Patients unrealistically may seek the breast form at a higher level on the chest and mistakenly believe that breast reduction procedure can achieve that. The base of the breast is where it is anatomically located and, if there is a degree of ptosis, that usually is adjusted during surgery, but it cannot reposition the base of the breast to a higher position. There should be a specific discussion in tall-chested patients about realistic results as well as a possibility of additional maneuvers to increase the upper pole, such as fat injections into the upper chest.[2] The entire area of patient expectations is fraught with misconceptions and challenges. The misunderstanding of being able to raise the base of the breast higher on the chest is an example of an incorrect patient expectation. Many patients believe that once a reduction occurs, any future level of ptosis will not occur. It is important to mention that their skin texture is unchanged and whatever genetic propensity for stretch and laxity they have will remain. I have discussed with my patients that bottoming out or relaxing the inferior pole can be common, and often an office procedure in the future to regain breast shape may be indicated.

SIZE AND SHAPE ARE ALWAYS AN ISSUE FOR THE PATIENT SEEKING BREAST REDUCTION

Breast asymmetry is not uncommon and should be addressed as well. Patients have an understanding of their own cup size, but that is dependent on which manufacturer's bra they wear. There is a wide diversity of size and manufacturers that can be confusing and bothersome to patients. The end result of a reduction, either too big or too small, is a main reason for litigation. Surgeons should spend the time to determine patient expectations and if they are achievable and realistic. See what bra size and manufacturer they are currently wearing and establish some realistic goals as to desired size and shape. Some manufacturers are designed to have their bras a larger cup than normal and others may be the opposite. If a desired cup size is documented, be sure to include the manufacturer. There is a big difference between a Victoria's Secret C cup and a Bali C cup. I emphasize a desired shape and whichever bra fits this desired shape may be more advantageous than a specific company. It is just as important to include measurements of the chest and breast sizes, which often demonstrate asymmetry and significant laxity. There are methods of breast displacement to help determine volume, although these are not statistical.

SYMMETRY

Although attempts are made to achieve symmetry, it is often difficult to adjust completely. Patients should be made aware of subtle differences between breasts as well as potential healing and swelling issues that may affect the final result. There are large-breasted patients who reach a point in their lives where they desire a significant reduction, often more than their overall frame and size dictate. Such demands should be a caution and a significant dialogue encouraged in an attempt to avoid an over-resection that patients then are unhappy with. This leads to one of the reasons liability has increased with breast reduction. The balance between a patient's goals and insurance coverage is a concern and a dilemma. There are patients who expect full coverage under their insurance yet want to remain a full appropriate shape for their size. There are charts available from most health care providers that indicate clear approval based on their own parameters, considering height, weight, and breast excision size. The gray area, the area listed in these charts that are not clearly accepted or rejected for size alone, must be approached cautiously. If a DDD cup patient is seeking improvement to a full C cup or small D cup, resulting in a 650-g excision, and the insurance requires a 1000-g excision, that is a problem. If a surgeon provides an excellent result at 650-g excision, the patient may be unhappy when the bills start coming after insurance denial. Conversely, if insurance coverage is approved for that 1000-g excision but the patient is unhappy being too small (small C cup) and not reaching expectations, who has been served? This insurance dilemma seems to be increasing. It may be that with increasing deductibles and co-pay requirements, an alternative may be a cosmetic procedure with known financial liabilities. If poor choices are made as to resection amounts and techniques, liability may result. Be cautious in the submission of authorization requests or when comments have been made to prospective patients by any member of the treatment team, especially seeking insurance coverage in a patient unable to become a self-pay patient. A free authorization letter is not a guarantee of coverage but can be used as a guide and honest excision amount. If the excision is overestimated, for instance, in the example where 650 g is expected to be excised but leading the insurance company to believe there is a 1000-g excision, the intent to deceive or confuse is considered fraud or abuse and may make the surgeon responsible for the failed outcome.[3,4]

Another alleged increase in litigation is due to newer techniques that are designed to limit scarring yet fail to achieve a satisfactory shape. This is a general and broad statement and must be adjusted to specifically meet patient goals and expectations. Patients with a large, ptotic breast who seek a reduction by liposuction may be happy with the minimal external scars but unhappy with the resulting shape. Similarly, those procedures that may promise to avoid a vertical scar are satisfactory as long as they do not compromise a resultant shape. Scarring is always an issue but lack of appropriate shape may be a bigger issue. The balance between achieving goals that are realistic and procedure choice is a critical one and should involve patient input. That is not to say that patients dictate procedure. I believe strongly that a patient cannot consent to what is believed to be a negligent procedure. The surgeon should protect a patient sometimes from the patient's own choice. Defendant physicians who claim this is what the patient wanted despite being forewarned about results may have a difficult assertion. There are always many options in achieving results but surgeons should help patients with choices that are safe and predictable. Sometimes such a safe and predictable result involves external scarring and the patient should understand that.

PATHOLOGY OF THE BREAST SPECIMEN

Pathology should be reviewed and a preoperative assessment of breast pathology and prior examinations should be sought. If there is a choice in breast reduction procedures, possibly an excision including questionable tissue may be achievable. For example, if a large pendulous 1500-g excision is planned for a 50-year-old woman with central calcifications that have been followed, a nipple graft procedure in which the central breast tissue can be removed and evaluated may have advantages. There may be strict limitations when this is possible; however, I have discovered many breast cancers in pathology specimens. All pathology specimens should be reviewed and a good practice pattern is to give patients a copy for their records.

REVISION POLICY–FINANCIAL POLICY

It is wise to have a revision policy and a financial policy that are disclosed to patients preoperatively. The revision policy describes the possibility of scar revision or adjustment in the future as long as a patient has been 100% compliant in postoperative care. The costs of surgeon, facility, and anesthesia should be discussed. Many risk managers recommend not charging for adjustment and revisions within the first year. There may be additional charges, however, for facility and anesthesia if the revision cannot be performed as an office procedure. Pathology costs should also be outlined. The financial policy should include possibilities of insurance denial; credit card challenges, including Health Insurance Portability and Accountability Act (HIPAA) release acknowledging their awareness of personal information protection while accepting the release of necessary personal health information as a response should the patient challenge credit card usage after treatment is provided; and overall estimates of costs and expenses. Patients may pay a portion or all of a surgeon's fees with a credit card, only to then challenge payment with the credit card company after surgery. HIPAA may prohibit a surgeon from discussing specifics of service provided without a release. The financial policy should include such a release if a challenge occurs.

PHOTOGRAPHS AND PATIENT PRIVACY

Photographs and patient privacy are new areas of concern. Photographs are required and usually sent to a managed care provider for preauthorization. Patients should consent to such photographs in a standard HIPAA consent. If the photographs are used, however, on a Web site, demonstration book in the office, or other commercial uses, a specific commercial HIPAA consent is required. The specific use of the photograph, the projected time span, and other details should be incorporated in the consent. In addition, the metadata stored within the digital photograph should be scrubbed or removed. Significant liability exists if no consent is obtained and patient private information is kept within a digital image and is discoverable.[5–8]

INFORMED CONSENT

The process of informed consent can be a lengthy one and is not fully reflected by the resulting document. It is difficult to achieve an understanding and completion of the informed consent process in 1 visit and then rapidly proceed to surgery. The duty of informed consent falls mainly on the surgeon but certainly can include a team effort. The key is to achieve an understanding of patient goals and expectations and attempt to match the procedure to predictably reach those goals. Surgeons should understand states' standard of informed consent, whether the reasonable physician standard or the reasonable patient standard. The reasonable distinction implies that information about the procedure, risks, hazards, alternatives, medications, and aftercare is explained and understood so that reasonable patients can make an informed decision or at a level that a reasonable physician would perform. I have always added a paragraph that the patient understands the risks, alternatives, and hazards as well as that no warrantees are created and further understanding what can and cannot be done the patient elects to proceed. The document is signed and witnessed but the process of achieving those is more important.

Breast reduction surgery is a most rewarding procedure for patients. Following some of these guidelines can help restore this surgery to the high satisfaction level it deserves and limit liability concerns.

REFERENCES

1. Gorney M. Avoiding litigation in breast modification. Plast Reconstr Surg 2011;127(5):2113–5.
2. Breast position on the chest wall. PSN, July-August 2013.
3. Beauty is skin deep – ugly to the bone. PSN, March 2013.
4. Gorney M. Ten years' experience in aesthetic surgery malpractice claims. Aesthet Surg J 2001;21(6): 569–71.
5. HIPAA Section 164.514(b)(2). Standards for Privacy of Individually Identifiable Health Information; Final Rule. 45 CFR Parts 160 and 164. Federal Register 65, no. 250 (December 28, 2000).
6. Scrub your commercial photographs.Plastic Surgery Pulse News; Vol. 7, Issue 2, 2015.
7. Gardner HE. Multiple intelligences: the theory in practice, a reader. Basic Books; 1993.
8. Mintz J, Wirshing DA. Informed consent: assessment of comprehension. Am J Psychiatry 1998;11(155): 1508–11.

FURTHER READINGS

Anderson RE. Medical malpractice: a physician's sourcebook. Humana Press Inc: Totowa (NJ); 2005.
Babe ruth syndrome. PSN, 2015.
Barrows RC Jr, Clayton PD. Privacy, confidentiality, and electronic medical records. J Am Med Inform Assoc 1996;3:139–48.
Barton HM. Medical records can win or lose a malpractice case. Tex Med 1990;86:33–6.
Berlin L. Alteration of medical records. AJR Am J Roentgenol 1997;168:1405–8.
Charles HT. Grabb and Smith's plastic surgery. 7th edition. Lippencott; 2013.
Choosing patients you like. PSN, July-August 2015.
EHR risk update. PSN, April-May 2014.
Gorney M, Martello J. Patient selection criteria. Clin Plast Surg 1999;26:37–40.
Haeck P, Gorney M. Electronic medical records may cast physicians in unfavorable light during lawsuits. Risk, liability and malpractice: what every plastic surgeon needs to know. Philadelphia: Saunders; 2011.
In search of normal expectations and return to attention to detail.
Jena AB, Seabury S, Lakdawalla D, et al. Malpractice risk according to physician specialty. N Engl J Med 2011;365(7):629–36.
Nahabedian MY. Plastic surgery beware. Plast Reconstr Surg 2014;133(4):965–6.
Nahai F, Reisman N. Pitfalls of online and digital communications with patients. Plastic Surgery News 2011; 129:5S.
Reisman N. On Legal Grounds. Plastic Surgery News.
Reisman N. Information that can and cannot be shared with colleagues. Plastic Surgery Pulse News 2013; 5:3.
Rinker B, Donnelly M, Henry C, et al. The standardized patient used for teaching patient selection in aesthetic surgery. Plastic Surgery News 2007;12553.
The ADA. PSN, October-November 2015.
Lane C. The distance learning technology resource guide, Multiple intelligences. Howard Gardner. (2010).
The electronic records information trap. PSN, September 2015.

Index

Note: Page numbers of article titles are in **boldface** type.

Clin Plastic Surg 43 (2016) 445–447
http://dx.doi.org/10.1016/S0094-1298(16)30008-6
0094-1298/16/$ – see front matter © 2016 Elsevier Inc. All rights reserved.

Moving?

Make sure your subscription moves with you!

To notify us of your new address, find your **Clinics Account Number** (located on your mailing label above your name), and contact customer service at:

Email: journalscustomerservice-usa@elsevier.com

800-654-2452 (subscribers in the U.S. & Canada)
314-447-8871 (subscribers outside of the U.S. & Canada)

Fax number: 314-447-8029

Elsevier Health Sciences Division
Subscription Customer Service
3251 Riverport Lane
Maryland Heights, MO 63043

*To ensure uninterrupted delivery of your subscription, please notify us at least 4 weeks in advance of move.

Printed and bound by CPI Group (UK) Ltd, Croydon, CR0 4YY

08/05/2025

01864682-0003